Demystifying Dog Behaviour for the Veterinarian is a ⸻ ⸻ ⸻ ⸻ ⸻ ⸻ designed to firstly help veterinarians understand their canine patients by seeing the world from the dog's perspective, and secondly how to safely and humanely handle them. Kendal debunks all the common detrimental myths on dog behaviour including the dreaded dominant dog concept. This well-referenced text is chock-full of practical tips and anecdotes from Kendal's wealth of case-studies (as a veterinarian, behaviour veterinarian and expert legal witness for the UK courts) to help the busy veterinary practitioner. A must read for all vets truly interested in safeguarding the welfare of the dog.

--Valerie Jonckheer-Sheehy, EBVS® European Veterinary Specialist in Behavioural Medicine, Head of Behaviour and Welfare IVC Evidensia, The Netherlands

The behaviour textbook that's been missing! An extremely valuable resource for the first opinion veterinary professional, at all stages of their career and training. Kendal provides welcomed illumination on this topic using a unique combination of shared life experiences from her perspectives as an early career vet, through to veterinary behaviourist and expert witness work, with case-based accounts, and references to just the right amount of theory. Essential tools are provided to aid vets in their canine observations and interactions, helping support their clients, and promote the mental health component of welfare. Although aimed at vets, this accessible text has many transferable messages and practical advice, and will appeal to a wider audience whose interest is in enhancing their canine understanding.

--Dr Mandy Roshier, Associate Professor in Anatomy and Behaviour, University of Nottingham, School of Veterinary Medicine and Science, UK

Demystifying Dog Behaviour for the Veterinarian not only reflects on best veterinary handling of dogs, but makes owners consider how they can help their dogs too. It's refreshing for the author to use references, but also acknowledge how the veterinarian's handling methods might change as their experience and understanding advances. Well worth a read!

--Chelsie Bailey, BSc Animal Behaviour & Welfare Science, UK

Kendal brings her wealth of experience as a veterinarian, clinical animal behaviourist and legal expert to this book, which is a must read highly accessible text for any veterinarian in general practice. The excellent use of illustrations, analogies and anecdotes leads the reader form the background of dog-human interactions, through to practical tips on managing dogs in veterinary practice. The inclusion of case reports provides contextual relevance to further add to the practical use of this book which will make any practitioner more behaviourally aware and thus improve the welfare of the dogs under our care.

--Kevin J. McPeake, BVMS PGDip(CABC) AFHEA MRCVS, Veterinary Behaviourist and Lecturer in Clinical Animal Behaviour, University of Edinburgh

DEMYSTIFYING DOG BEHAVIOUR FOR THE VETERINARIAN

Kendal Shepherd

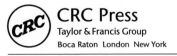

CRC Press
Taylor & Francis Group
Boca Raton London New York

CRC Press is an imprint of the
Taylor & Francis Group, an **informa** business

Photographs copyright Kendal Shepherd unless otherwise noted.

First edition published 2021
by CRC Press
6000 Broken Sound Parkway NW, Suite 300, Boca Raton, FL 33487-2742

and by CRC Press
2 Park Square, Milton Park, Abingdon, Oxon, OX14 4RN

© 2021 Taylor & Francis Group, LLC

CRC Press is an imprint of Taylor & Francis Group, LLC

Library of Congress Cataloging-in-Publication Data

ISBN: 978-0-367-71639-4 (hbk)
ISBN: 978-0-367-54991-6 (pbk)
ISBN: 978-1-003-15303-0 (ebk)

Typeset in Times
by MPS Limited, Dehradun

Contents

Foreword

Why am I writing this book?

Well, first of all because I was asked to. In January 2018, I gave a presentation entitled, 'What has behaviour got to do with welfare assessment?' at the British Veterinary Forensics and Law Association winter meeting. Using welfare legal cases involving dogs in which I'd provided evidence for the Defence, I illustrated how vital it was to be able to assess a dog's behaviour in order to give an opinion about welfare state of those alleged to have suffered. Unbeknownst to me at the time, the meeting was attended by the delightful Alice Oven of Taylor & Francis publishers. Sometime after the meeting, I received an email from her wondering would I be interested in writing a book for veterinarians (rather than veterinary surgeons, it being intended for worldwide readership) and could I put together a proposal for review?

Flattered as I was by this invitation, I couldn't help but wonder what possible interest a well-known publisher of academic literature had in me. If anyone embodied the art rather than the science of veterinary medicine, I was that person. After all, when pleading to be allowed to resit my fourth year at Bristol, having yet again failed the requisite exams, I was asked in all seriousness, 'Are you sure you wouldn't rather be an actress, Miss Kirkland?' I realised then that the spectre of a brief dalliance with the university Drama Society, evidence of which first emerged in my first year, still cast its prejudicial shadow over my reputation. After only the briefest of hesitations and in the knowledge that it would be far easier to imagine acting, rather than vetting, as a hobby, I gave a sufficiently emphatic 'Yes – I want to be a vet!'.

Spurred on by Alice's invitation and enthusiastic reviews of the proposal, her subsequent cajoling over nearly two years paid off. Aided and abetted by a personal disaster (a stroke) and a social one (the COVID-19 pandemic), I have eventually had the time to commit 'pen to paper'. This is the result.

Author

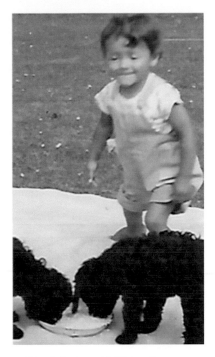

Kendal circa 1955 aged two.

Dr. Kendal Shepherd, BVSc., MRCVS, qualified from Bristol University in 1978. With extensive experience in small animal practice, she was the first veterinary surgeon to be accredited by ASAB as a certificate clinical animal behaviourist in 2005. She is heavily involved in the behavioural assessment of dogs under both sections 1 and 3 of the Dangerous Dogs Act 1991 and also accepts instruction in welfare cases. Her particular interests are: promoting the need for vet/medic co-operation in thorough and expert investigation of all dog bite incidents, including fatalities, the routine education of children regarding dog bite prevention; and the encouragement of all veterinary professionals to routinely safeguard the behaviour of their patients in all the cases that they treat.

Kendal's family was never without pets, including a variety of dogs. Her earliest memory is of multiple poodle puppies bred by her mother whereas later during her school years, she fondly remembers the Siamese cat which dropped all her kittens behind the piano, a litter of hamsters revived by a neighbour's timely administration of drops of brandy, the tortoise awaking after hibernation with only three legs and an afternoon ostensibly out blackberrying but actually spent rescuing a mongrel puppy stuck down a rabbit warren, with the help of local gypsies. The salamanders, stick insects, guinea pigs, and budgerigars together with a variety of cats provided at times a veritable home-spun food chain.

Acknowledgement

There are so many people (and dogs) who have helped me in their various ways to my current understanding. This does not mean that I have always agreed with what I've read or been told but even disagreements can be both instructive and constructive. A few are mentioned by name and referenced in this book – Ian Dunbar, Turid Rugaas, Danny Mills, Roger Mugford, Myrna Milani, John Bradshaw and James Serpell – but please take this as a very big thankyou to all those I've ever come across in the context of vetting and dogs. I must specifically thank the wonderful artist, Victor Ambrus and his wife, Glenys. I was lucky enough to have his illustrations accompany the text of the Canine Commandments and he has given permission for them to be reproduced here. His intuitive understanding and visual interpretation of what I was trying to say in the text was perfect.

This book is dedicated to the memory of my mother from whom I have obviously inherited the inability to live without dogs.

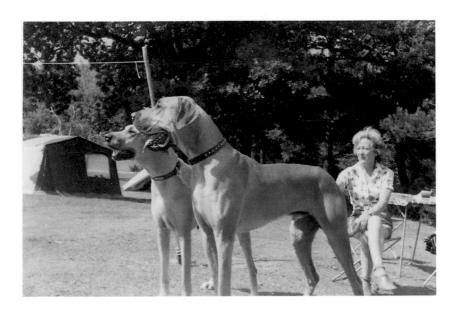

Introduction

It is said that dogs, as people, are a product of nature and, of equal importance, nurture. Nurture encompasses everything a dog experiences, whether good or bad, intentional or not, in the name of dog training or simply hearing the vacuum cleaner or a thunderstorm for the first time. These experiences are never more important than during the 'socialisation period' (from 6 to 14 weeks), during which the puppy brain is at its most plastic and able to respond accordingly. Neural pathways and, in turn, emotional responses are formed for better or worse. Such responses and attendant behaviour, desirable or not, will become fixed in the canine behavioural repertoire. The more opportunity for rehearsal, as with piano scales, the better 'fixed' in the repertoire the behaviour will be.

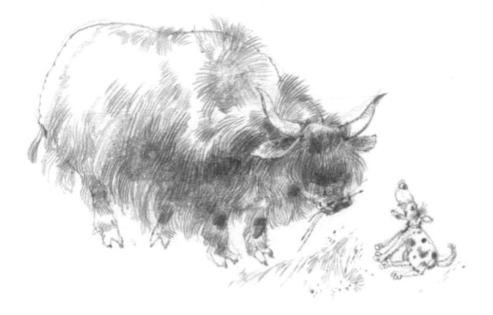

Illustration by Victor Ambrus.

It is therefore critical that such lessons result, as far as possible, in behaviour patterns which will be acceptable to people and fully equip the young dog to deal appropriately with everything it may encounter later in life.

Unfortunately, this is not always the case. Puppies bred for appearance rather than healthy bodies and sound temperament continue to present at best unpromising and at worst pathological material with which to begin. Completely foreseeable behaviours are often condoned by family and friends in a puppy's 'formative years' – house soiling, jumping up, pulling on lead, and of course aggression ('he didn't mean it', 'it was only a nip') – and there may be an ill-based assumption that the puppy will 'grow out of it'. The result is that well-rehearsed behaviours are later identified as 'problems' and need 'treatment' in adulthood. It is not an exaggeration to state that, if such behaviours impact on people sufficiently, they are as life-threatening as any conventional disease.

Canine aggression is the predominant issue in all people's minds, not least for veterinary surgeons, who may not only fear for their own safety but are also professionally obliged to keep their staff as well as their clients in one piece. Sadly, despite the best of intentions, the means by which this is achieved may teach the young dog that the surgery is a place to be feared rather than enjoyed. All too common misunderstandings regarding the purpose of canine aggression result in ill-advised reprimand and coercive handling. The result? Behaviour which is not only dangerous but potentially illegal.

I therefore make no apologies for laying the blame, at least in part, for such early behavioural damage fairly and squarely at the veterinary door. Crimes of omission may have as damaging consequences as those of commission. Failure to personally check out the credentials and abilities of the dog trainer whose business card has been pinned without question to the waiting room notice board and to whom vulnerable young puppies are duly sent for their 'education' may have untoward consequences. Equally, indelible memories of pain and fear may be accidentally instilled at first vaccination, causing permanent damage if handled poorly. Faulty lessons learned in the surgery or puppy class spread, like infection, into other real-life contexts.

In my experience, while going back in a dog's history during a behaviour consultation for aggression, or when preparing for a legal instruction regarding a dog which has bitten, it is not uncommon to find a salient moment in a dog's veterinary career when a seismic shift in a young canine patient's perception of the world occurred. If previously hopeful and trusting – a 'pint half full' optimistic dog – the world suddenly seemed to become hostile and uncaring, so that more than a modicum of wariness was to be required in the future. If the metaphorical pint was already half empty, then one's worst fears were simply confirmed.

Such incidents may appear at the time to be inconsequential, but oh-so-commonly-heard phrases such as 'he knows where he is!' or 'my last dog didn't like the vets either!' must be taken for what they really mean rather than being simply a cue for polite laughter. The interpretation should be 'my dog is afraid and needs urgent help or he may bite in the future'. Nor should the panting, bouncy patient dragging his owner through the door with furiously wagging tail be taken at face value as a dog who 'loves being here!' Does he really love the surgery or are these symptoms of a highly stressed animal desperately in need of behavioural guidance? Treating the lame or vomiting dog may be easily accomplished; reversing behavioural damage is not.

So what does this little book hope to achieve? Vets have so much on their plate already and seem assailed by pressures to learn ever-increasing amounts. Continuing Professional Development (CPD) looms large even for new graduates. They may have hardly found their way round the consulting room, let alone their feet in the wider world of general veterinary practise, before the obligation to 'continue their professional development' is thrust upon them.

The problem, as I see it, is that historically, the behavioural sphere, unlike any other, was launched onto the veterinary profession as a fully formed speciality rather than growing organically out of general practise first. As such, texts generally available to veterinary surgeons were, and still are, heavily referenced tomes, befitting such specialism. Without digesting the whole, how were busy vets and nurses to educate themselves in humanely extricating a kennel guarding dog from its hospital cage or give a fractious animal a vaccination? One may be able to get the job done by time-honoured and expedient means, but have we been storing up trouble for the future, not only for the surgery but for the world at large?

The intention is not to preach to the choir, not to create more 'specialists', nor berate those who have not appreciated the need for a more enlightened behavioural approach to the canine patient. There will be little by way of theory of this or that nor indeed any long words at all – simply practical advice supplemented with analogies and educational anecdotes to be used by both client and attending veterinary surgeon to improve a dog's view of life in general, as well as of the surgery specifically. As painlessly as possible, and maybe without being aware of it all, a little theory may well sink in.

Above all, I will encourage all readers to routinely and actively demonstrate how to handle and communicate with dogs while becoming better aware of the behavioural impact of all veterinary procedures. This will enhance the relationship of the patient and client with the surgery as well as make life safer for everyone. In other words, the message to clients must become not just 'Do as I say', but 'Do as I do'. There is no better way to turn theory into practise for the benefit and welfare of all concerned.

With this in mind, and with no further ado, I will begin with what being a dog actually entails, followed closely by the dos and don'ts of the behaviourally aware practitioner.

Part I

Dogs and vets

1 What is a dog?

It has often occurred to me that although they have a Latin name, *Canis familiaris*, we have generally never thought of the pet dog as a species at all. Dogs are so inextricably and uniquely involved with humans that we do not consider their habitat, ecology and environment in the same way one would, for example, that of the kangaroo, whale, elephant or red kite. It is as if the dog has come to be viewed as a human accoutrement only, to be used and, dare I say, abused, according to human needs only. After all, the domestic dog is hardly an endangered species, far from it. With an estimated 470 million pet dogs worldwide, with perhaps 900 million free-ranging or human satellite dogs, it is arguably the most successful of creatures, with no need for protection or special concern. It is only relatively recently that the domestic dog in all its myriad of shapes and sizes has generated any science of its own, rather than being assumed to be an offshoot of the grey wolf, physically different but with behavioural traits intact. But the question is: how correct have we been in our conclusions about the social structure and behaviour of the wolf in the first place? And then how correct have we been when we began to apply the same assumed rules to the dog?

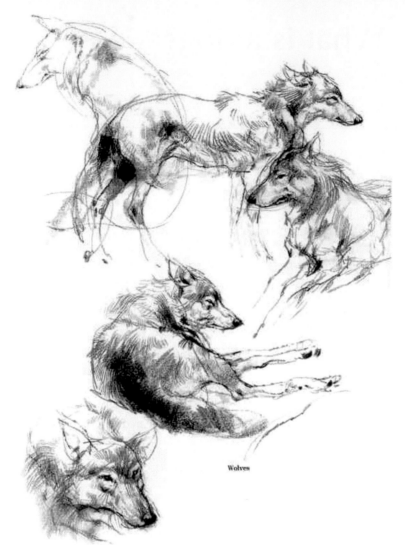

Wolves

Illustration by Victor Ambrus.

When fighting for our own share of the duvet or hoping that Fido won't actually bite the postman, we tend to forget dogs' historic use as a hot water bottle or as guardian of property. Have we contributed to the evolutionary double bind the dog now finds itself in?

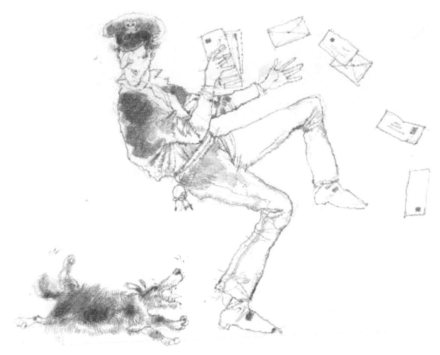

Illustration by Victor Ambrus.

So why do we get along with dogs and why don't we? It has to be said that as a species, *Homo sapiens* seems to have a rather schizophrenic attitude towards animals in general, and dogs in particular. As epitomised in Hal Herzog's book *Some We Love, Some We Hate and Some We Like to Eat*, the domestic dog can, in certain circumstances and cultures, fall into all three categories. In the UK alone, the dog is all at once 'man's best friend' and a creature which can, in the blink of an eye, turn so savage as to put life and limb at risk.

Much has been postulated and fairly confidently written about the origins of the domestic dog as a species, but the jury still seems to be out on exactly when and where the transformation from wild canid to cuddly pet began. There is pretty much agreement that the dog and modern-day wolf had a common ancestor and that this animal was predisposed to selective pressure. This pressure was imposed mainly accidentally, by aspects of the lifestyle and propensities that humans and wolves have in common.

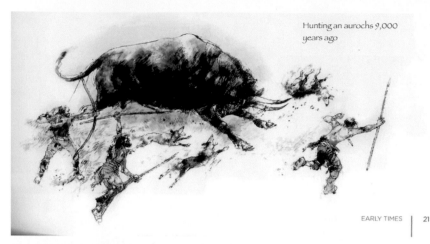

Cooperative hunting: hunting an aurochs 9000 years ago. Image by Victor Ambrus, reproduced with permission from the South West Heritage Trust.

The 'successful scavenger' is a concept, proposed by Ray Coppinger in 2001, which encompasses the human tendency for indiscriminate disposal of waste, the opportunistic feeding habits of the wolf and the accidental selection for tameness which would have resulted. Those individuals among the wolf population which were least afraid of man had the greatest chances of success.

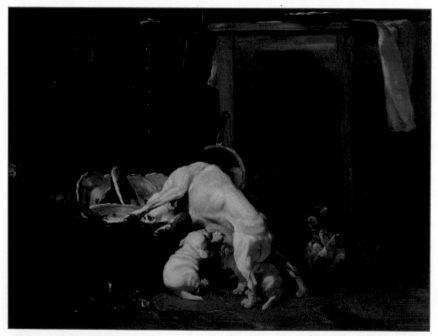

'Everyone for himself' (Chacun Pour Soi), Philippe Rousseau, 1864.

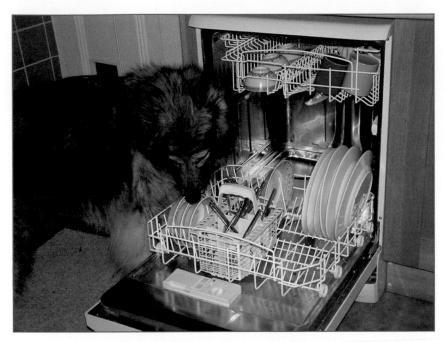

Modern-day equivalent of 'the successful scavenger'?

The experimental selection for tameness as a behavioural trait in silver foxes began in the Institute of Cytology and Genetics in Novosibirsk, Siberia, (Belyaev 1959 onwards) and seemed to have accounted solely for dog-like physical changes, such as having floppy tails and ears, variation in coat colour, bi-annual seasons and smaller brains. But selection for this trait of tameness alone has recently been questioned (Lord et al. 2020). Other genetic selection, such as for the ability to digest starch, may have also favoured those animals scavenging human waste, part of the domestication syndrome. Add to this the culture-wide and historic human trait of pet-keeping, whereby a young wild animal is adopted and effectively tamed, a genetic pool is formed from which a truly domesticated species may emerge.

There is evidence that a similar process is happening among red foxes in urban environments today. Having been struck by how fearless these foxes appeared as they strolled between rubbish bins, Kevin Parsons of Glasgow University studied fox skulls collected from London and adjacent countryside between 1971 to 1973 (royalsocietypublishing.org/journal/rspb). The skull shapes varied significantly between habitats. The urban foxes, like their Russian counterparts, had developed shorter and wider muzzles, seemingly favouring a stronger bite over the need for speed, which would be provided by a more slim-line shape.

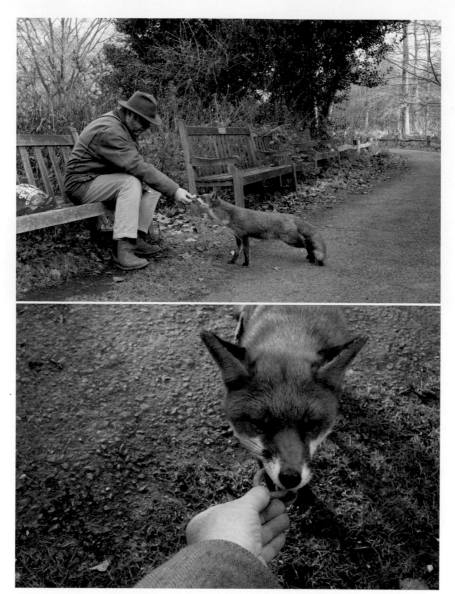

Domestication in progress, courtesy Solent News.

Ultimately, once the vagaries of human taste and preference for appearance were also brought to bear, this amalgam of selection for behaviour, looks and ability resulted in the variety of canine shapes and sizes we see today. These variations however are definitely not all to the dog's advantage, either as a species or as an individual, as will be discussed later.

But it is the fact that wolves were social and lived in groups that is the most relevant for my purpose. Of necessity a means of communication was required which limited the need and desire to kill each other. The communication whereby wolves, and their descendants dogs, manage this, to my mind, provides both the reason for the domestic dog's success and, paradoxically, its downfall. It has created the dichotomy faced by today's dogs.

To understand this, it is essential to correct erroneous but persistent beliefs in the social structure of wolves and how it is maintained. Early studies of wolf behaviour were carried out largely on captive animals – disparate groups of unrelated wolves of varying age and sex thrown together in limited space. In such inevitably stressed animals, a completely false impression was created of a society in which aggression seemed to be the main form of communication. Individuals were labelled as to how aggressive they were in encounters and the most successful (possibly daring) were considered dominant to the submissive losers. Far from communication serving the purpose of reducing stress and strife in social animals, it was assumed that every individual was simply waiting for any opportunity to gain aggressive advantage over its companions. Furthermore, any individual who reached the top of pecking order had to watch his back continually for any aggressive challengers, a form of canid *coup d'etat*.

Studies of wolves more recently released into the wild, specifically into Yellowstone Park USA in 1995, revealed just how wrong this notion was (www.yellowstonepark.com). Free-ranging wolves were observed to form co-operative family groups, just as people. Squabbles only rarely broke out, therefore requiring an urgent re-evaluation of how peaceful communication was achieved. The parents of such families had had the fictitious 'alpha' or 'dominant' status assigned to them simply because they did what parents do everywhere – educate and, if necessary, discipline any unruly offspring. Once maturity was reached, young adults might decide to leave the family group and set up on their own, again not unlike human families.

One of the first to acknowledge the mistake he had made in interpreting wolf social behaviour in his influential book *The Wolf: Ecology and Behavior of an Endangered Species*, published in 1970, was ecologist L. David Mech (www.davidmech.org/wolf news). In his article 'Whatever happened to the term "alpha wolf"?', published in the winter of 2008 in the *International Wolf* journal, he states,

Most other general wolf books have relied considerably on 'The Wolf' for information, thus spreading the misinformation about alpha wolves far and wide.

Rather than viewing a wolf pack as a group of animals organised with a 'top dog' that fought its way to the top, or a male-female pair of such aggressive wolves, science has come to understand that most wolf packs are merely family groups formed in exactly the same way as human families are formed. (p. 7)

But there had been many previous decades for the dominance myth to infiltrate the world of the domestic and pet dog. Dogs were thought to need dominating by their human companions to keep them in their place and prevent a 'take-over bid'. Moreover, this had to be achieved by coercive and downright violent means.

Unfortunately, to the detriment of dogs and owners everywhere, this erroneous notion was taken up avidly by certain elements of the dog training world, particularly those of a military bent, well-schooled in fighting to win. The methods advocated by Colonel Konrad Most in his 1910 book, *Dog Training: A Manual* were of this ilk, as are the various far more recent publications by The Monks of New Skete. Titles such as 'How to be your dog's best friend' belie the aggressive way this relationship is advised to be forged, if anything serving only to seriously damage the mutual trust evolution had created.

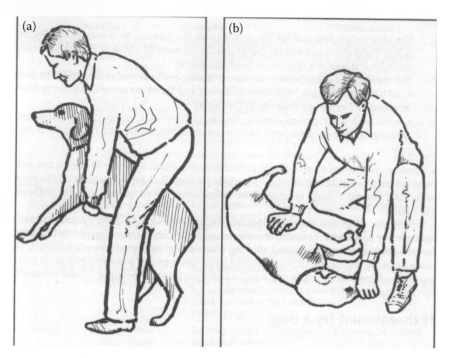

'Dominant but fair' dominance exercises

Doglopaedia 1997

Commonly advised ways to assert 'dominance' over a dog have been to hold a dog up by the scruff of the neck or, as illustrated, under the chest, or to pin a dog down to the floor by the muzzle. I have come across veterinary surgeons who have demonstrated this supposed means of putting a dog in its place, when faced with an unruly puppy in consultation. In reality, nothing is more guaranteed to teach pre-emptive aggression in adulthood. There seems little point in vaccinating against fatal infectious disease if, at the same time, one is causing potentially fatal behavioural damage.

Times and attitudes are however changing, albeit slowly, and not soon enough to salvage many broken relationships evidenced by rehoming centres becoming full to capacity. In spite of studies which have shown that coercive and threatening training methods are associated with aggressive responses in dogs (e.g., Casey et al. 2014), practise has not caught up with theory and dog owners are still urged by books, the media and certain dog trainers to be 'leaders of the pack'. Their pet must be left in no doubt of where they stand in the hierarchy. Only a few weeks ago I received the veterinary history of a young male Jack Russell aggressive towards his owners who was described as having 'dominance issues' in his notes. Along with the earth's supposed position at the centre of the solar system and the Flat Earth Society, such beliefs must be consigned to history for the welfare and sanity of our canine companions.

Differences between wolves and dogs

Wolves
> Extended family groups
> Cooperative hunting
> Intolerant of wolves outside family group
> Intolerant of people
> Adults less playful than cubs

Dogs
> Groups of disparate heritage
> 'Selfish scavenger'
> Tolerant of unknown dogs
> Tolerant of unknown people
> Retention of puppy-like behaviour into adulthood

BUT … both species have a **common body language** which allows for harmonious group living. Moreover, during the course of evolution and adaptation to living in close proximity to people, dogs have become adept at **interpreting human gestures and expression**. Of great importance is to understand that the dog-human relationship developed throughout **without our deliberate interference**. We are only just beginning to unravel the influences, including on human behaviour, by which domestication occurred. Unless the dog is understood for what it really is, to the best of current knowledge, the unique relationship that exists between our species will be fatally damaged.

THE DEATH OF DOMINANCE

What is the appearance of a dog allegedly trying to be 'dominant'? Or, of equal importance, what does a dog look like when being 'submissive'? Do the terms dominance and submission have any real relevance to internal mental state of the individual dog or are they simply descriptions of appearance? To ascribe intent to an appearance is fraught with difficulty, and historically ethologists have assumed intent by observing the results of interactions between two individuals (or dyads). If the apparently dominant animal wins and the apparently submissive dog loses, then this is what must have been the outcome intended by each party. The terms thus became self-fulfilling prophecies.

The definition provided in 1993 by Drews states the following:

A dominance relationship can only exist **between two individuals** and is the result of repeated, agnostic interactions between them, characterised by a **consistent outcome** in favour of one individual and a **default yielding response** of the other rather than an escalation of aggression. The status of the consistent winner is dominant to the loser, who is subordinate. (p. 283)

If we have to mention it at all, dominance therefore:

1. Describes a relationship, not an individual animal
2. Is based on experience and mutual assessment of strengths and weaknesses and on-going cost-benefit analysis
3. Is context-specific with regard to resource value and expectation
4. Action of the deferent party determines the outcome of the interaction and confers dominance by default
5. **Serves to eliminate the need for aggression**

What, therefore, is the behaviour which determines the outcome of a supposed battle? Arguments are 'won' more by one side conceding defeat than being forcefully overcome, and it has been argued that the same is true for animals (Rowell 1974). If this is what is happening, contrary to popular belief, it is the actions of the deferent ('subordinate'/'submissive') dog which determines the nature of the relationship and most importantly the expectations of each party. It is when the customary expectation is confounded that instability in any relationship arises. The significance for the dog-human relationship is that we do not have to assume that dogs are forever trying to take advantage of us by aggressive means. It also means that, in order to accurately predict outcomes of interactions between individuals, there needs to be a reasonable degree of stability in the relationship. The reliability of body language and expression in achieving a desired outcome in the other party is what a stable relationship depends upon. Conversely, it is when the habitual provisions of one half of a relationship are at odds with the expectations of the other that disharmony results.

Dogs express their needs and desires in some very obvious ways which are difficult to misinterpret. The dog wagging a tail on being shown a dog lead can fairly safely be assumed to want to go for a walk as can the licking of lips and gazing in the direction of a food bowl show a desire to eat. But they also do it in far more subtle ways. Although more open to misinterpretation, these expressions have also been of huge benefit to dogs and humans have been more than willing participants in this process. How do they do it? A continuum of social gestures, variously termed 'calming signals' (Rugaas 1997), affiliative behaviour and threat aversion can all be placed under the umbrella term of appeasement behaviour. These have conspired together, I would suggest, to give rise to three overriding categories of canine appearance which, I would further suggest, have been largely responsible for the huge success of dogs. But at the same time, this success may be eroded as the appearances feed erroneous and damaging beliefs and management methods.

It is imperative to remember that, from the canine perspective, whatever differing intents assigned to these appearances by humans, they have only one expectation as to result. Which is calmness and the restoration of harmony.

These appearances are the following:

THE 'I LOVE YOU' LOOK

Just as Helen's face launched a thousand Greek ships towards ill-fated Troy, so did the 'I love you' look launch innumerable proto-dogs into the unique position they hold in human affection today. The doleful eyes, the laid-back ears, the licking of face and hands and the obvious delight they show after even the briefest of separations convince us of their undying and unconditional love.

Without wishing to spoil this illusion, this appearance has its origin in care-soliciting and appeasing behaviours shown by wolf cubs towards their mother. Current dog owners may not wish to be informed that the 'kisses' so willingly given were intended originally to stimulate regurgitation of food upon which the cubs could feed.

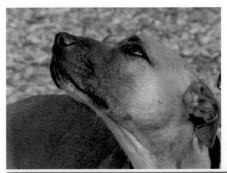

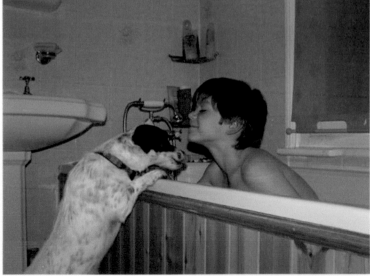

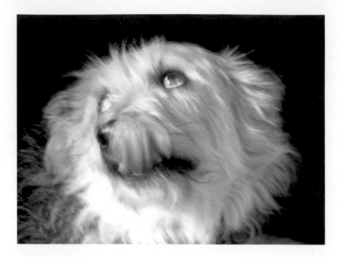

THE 'OBEDIENT' LOOK

So, too can the obedience of dogs be misleading in how it is interpreted by people. How has obedience been instilled and what is the canine response? If a dog is coerced into sitting or lying down, could our success in achieving the desired response be based on an innate expression of appeasement behaviour and mislead us into assuming a dog's understanding and therefore compliance? Is the dog 'giving paw' in the waiting room really doing something he's been trained to do or saying 'please let's go home'?

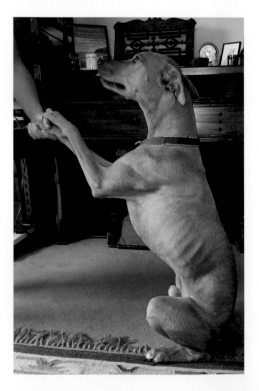

Interestingly, in the book *If Dogs Could Talk* (Csányi 2006), the author summarises how the modern dog was selected thus, 'Wolves or early dogs that attacked humans were killed, and hence the selection was accomplished; the result was a complaisant, trustworthy dog, **capable of being disciplined**'.

What allows the dog to tolerate 'discipline'? Could it be the strength of thousands of years of selection for appeasement behaviour and the benefits this brought to the species?

Appeasement behaviour, despite all its advantages, has also provided justification of coercive, dominance-based training methods: in a nutshell, 'Behave or I'll hit ya!'

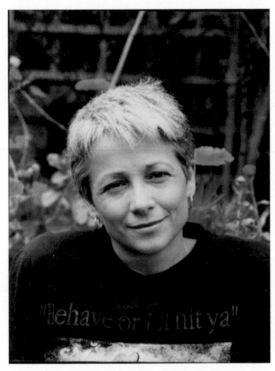

(see Ladder of Aggression, Chapter 5)

THE 'GUILTY' LOOK

How often have you heard that a dog 'knows he's done wrong' and therefore deserves our displeasure? But like the chicken and the egg, which comes first?

Studies have shown that dogs respond, not according to what they know they have done, but according to what their owners *think* their dog has done. A study carried out in 2009 (Horowitz) concluded that, if led to believe their dog had disobeyed instructions by stealing food in their absence, and the owner assumed an admonishing attitude on their return, then, *and only then*, did dogs assume an aura of guilt. This study however still did not entirely eliminate other evidence of wrongdoing, such as missing food, which could also have led a dog to assume the 'guilty look'. A further study in 2015 (Ostojic et al.) clarified that whether a dog had indeed stolen food in the owner's absence or not, it was human displeasure alone, and subsequent scolding, which triggered the 'guilty' look, rather than canine acknowledgement of guilt prompting the reprimand. Normal 'happy' greeting behaviour continued until the owner's attitude unexpectedly changed.

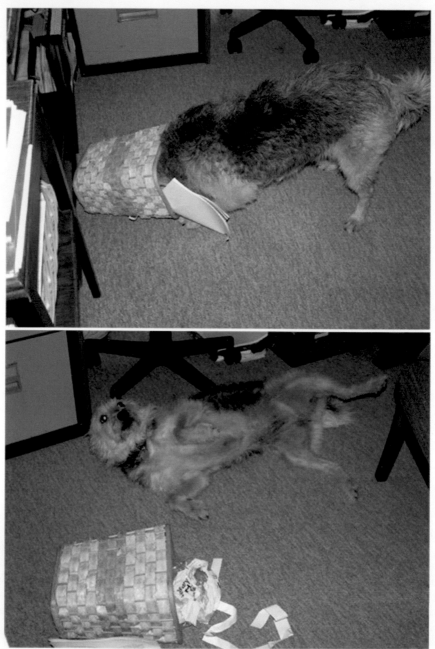

The purpose of the 'guilty' look? To immediately appease us and dissipate our anger. We accept the apparently heartfelt 'apology', even feeling sorry for the craven culprit, telling ourselves that he didn't really mean to upset us, and forgive them. Harmony is restored.

Until that is, the dog comes to realise that, despite his best efforts to pacify and calm, either during one episode or over a period of time, he is not being successful, the time for appeasement is over, and more overt means of repelling the threat posed has come.

THE STORY OF GELERT

The following is inscribed on a dog's gravestone in Beddgelert in Wales:

In the 13th century Llywelyn, prince of North Wales, had a palace at Beddgelert. One day he went hunting without Gelert, 'The Faithful Hound', who was unaccountably absent. On Llywelyn's return the truant, stained and smeared with blood, joyfully sprang to meet his master. The prince alarmed hastened to find his son, and saw the infant's cot empty, the bedclothes and floor covered with blood. The frantic father plunged his sword into the hound's side, thinking it had killed his heir. The dog's dying yell was answered by a child's cry. Llywelyn searched and discovered his boy unharmed, but nearby lay the body of a mighty wolf which Gelert had slain. The prince filled with remorse is said never to have smiled again. He buried Gelert here.

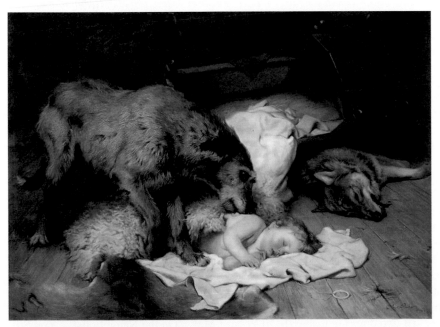

'Gelert', Charles Burton Barber, 1884.

So what actually happened? Imagine the scene.

On his master's return, Gelert was full of joy to see him, springing to greet him displaying canine greeting behaviour we would all recognise. No hint of guilt or acknowledgement of wrongdoing then. What changed? The prince became alarmed, the inscription informs us. Gelert, however, would surely have expected his customary friendly reciprocal greeting instead of alarm. His instant response was to attempt to calm his master, to appease, to restore equilibrium. His appearance can be visualised—ears back, crouched stance with tail tucked under, perhaps a hint of turning his head and body away from this unsettling reaction. In other words, plain admission of guilt. Stained with blood as he was, adding circumstantial evidence of criminal activity to this visual confession, Prince Llewellyn could draw no other conclusion. Guilty as charged.

Dogs are still dying owing to misinterpretation of the 'guilty' look. All it takes is the almost ubiquitous belief that dogs 'know they've done wrong' and the consequent and chronic punishment of the 'guilty' look for a dog to come to believe that overt aggression is the only thing that we understand.

However, looking 'guilty' can also soften the hardest of human hearts and has become a vital amalgam of gestures for any dog when faced with imminent human anger. If such appeasement behaviour has the intended result, that of mollifying a person, it will be reinforced and repeated.

KATE AND SAM

Many years ago I owned two dogs – Kate, a rather lovely looking German Shepherd cross Ibizan hound, and Sam, a good old-fashioned mongrel. Although generally well-behaved dogs, their only crime was to raid the rubbish bin every so often.

In the style of the true believer in canine guilt, I routinely directed my not-inconsiderable ire towards the grovelling hound, Kate, interpreting her behaviour as an abject apology for a repeated misdemeanour.

Until that is, one day when, on hearing a kerfuffle in the kitchen, the same dog ran in to the room apparently apologising for her behaviour in advance. Sam then nonchalantly walked in, butter unmelted in the mouth, with the lid of the kitchen swing-bin still dangling around his neck.

DOG SHAMING

There is currently a social media-fuelled fad for 'dog shaming'. This entails taking photographs of guilty-looking dogs, surrounded with evidence of their 'crime'. To add to their shame, details of their supposed 'confession' are placed around their neck, much as used to happen to convicted criminals on their way to the gallows. One needs to look no further for ultimate expressions of appeasement behaviour than these images of craven canines. There is even a dog shaming calendar featuring 'the best of canine shame fame'. Monthly captions such as 'Partners in Crime' (if two dogs are featured), 'It Wasn't Me!', 'On the Naughty list',' You Still Love Me, Right?' and 'I'm Lucky I'm Cute' proclaim both the fallacy and the inadvertent truth of the foundation of the human-canine relationship. With the presumed purpose of amusing the masses, it may serve to mislead instead.

(www.dogshaming.com)

THE DEPICTION OF DOGS IN ART

It seems that anthropomorphic projection of emotions and motives onto the animals we care for and are dependent upon, has, during the course of evolution and domestication, enabled us better to manipulate these animals to mutual benefit (Serpell 2002). Overall, anthropomorphism would therefore appear to be a valuable and adaptive trait, regardless of whether our assumptions are strictly accurate. However, misplacement of human values, motives and emotions onto dogs may also have disastrous consequences.

Art of many forms can be used as an illustration of the incorporation of anthropomorphism into human culture as it applies to animals in general and the domestic dog in particular. Words and phrases describing the emotions and motives assigned to dogs abound in all media, from classic breed descriptions in Kennel Club texts, to books, cartoons and animations, advertising, greetings cards, and in the replies of owners when questioned about their own individual dogs. 'Loyalty', 'fidelity', 'unconditional love and affection', 'protectiveness', 'bravery', 'jealousy', 'guilt', being 'biddable' and having the desire to 'please' are all descriptions and phrases used with little, if any, correlation with what a dog might actually be doing, look like or really want out of a situation, when thus described.

In *Expressions of the Emotions in Man and Animals*, Darwin proposes three principles to explain the physical expression of emotions: namely, 'serviceable habits', body postures which are found initially to be useful, therefore perpetuated as habits; 'antithesis', whereby opposing emotions are automatically accompanied by opposite physical appearances; and by the 'direct action of an excited nervous system'. Although recognising that intercommunication is of the highest importance in social animals and that emotions are clearly expressed in body postures and gestures, the actions themselves are thought frequently to offer no 'direct service' to the animal itself, and, this being the case, there seems to be little, if any, discussion as to their possible adaptive value.

But Darwin fell equally under the influence of anthropomorphism, interpreting body postures as signifying a 'humble and affectionate frame of mind', wanting to 'caress' his master and the assumed abject admission of 'Behold, I am your slave.' Was he correct in assuming the gestures were of no direct service to dogs? I would argue to the contrary – that the ability to appease us, and what such behaviour looks like, is the lynchpin upon which the dog-human relationship was founded.

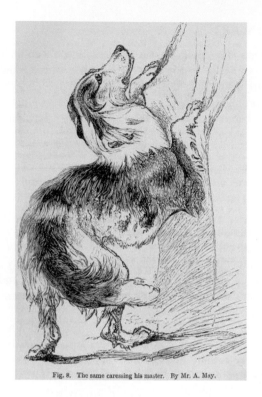

Fig. 8. The same caressing his master. By Mr. A. May.

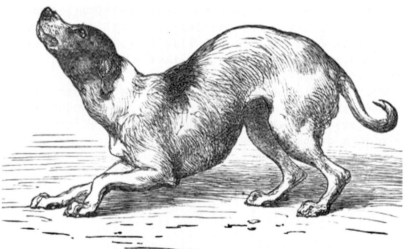

FIG. 6.—The same in a humble and affectionate frame of mind. By Mr. Riviere.

Visual art, as opposed to Darwin's early science, works by giving us a bodily image of a dog in a particular context, but leaving the observer to ascribe purpose and meaning to its actions and the possible reasons for its inclusion in the picture in the first place. Prior to the Victorian era, the presence of a dog at a marriage ceremony, for example, might be used to symbolise faithfulness and eternal love between two people, whereas in later works, the title of a painting, such as 'The Special Pleader', may hint at the artist's personal interpretation of the animal's own state of mind. The term 'special pleader' describes a lawyer who makes pleas of mitigation on behalf of his guilty client. One is left in no doubt therefore that in this case the dog is fulfilling this role on behalf of the child in distress.

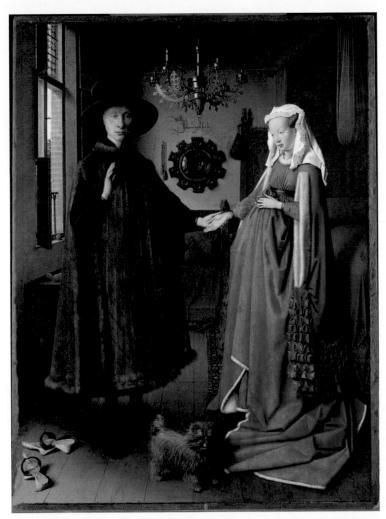

The Arnolfini portrait, Jan van Eyck, 1434.

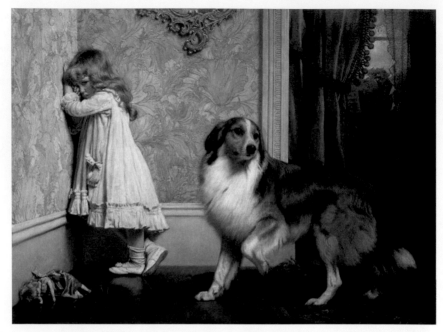

A Special Pleader, Charles Burton Barber, 1893.

But how accurate are these, or those of any later observers and commentators, and how might such interpretations colour our expectation of dogs, and hence our relationship with them?

Dogs are judged as to how far they appear to meet, or fall short of, human expectations. The beliefs perpetuated in art and literature inevitably affect our perception of the behaviour of dogs and in turn our view of its acceptability. They underpin the human view of dogs in all walks of life and will inform, rightly or wrongly, all decisions taken about dogs – for example, to approach or leave alone, to pet or reprimand or to keep or relinquish. A 'protective' dog may have been considered a boon to mankind for centuries, but what of the present-day magistrate presiding over a case of dog-human aggression? Will he or she be unusually immune to the belief that all dogs should want to please rather than bite us? Or will they instead be similarly prejudiced by cultural assumption and euphemism? The contribution of popular art to the perpetuation of these destructive myths cannot be underestimated.

Clarifying a dog's intentions as expressed in its body language is of crucial importance when counselling the owners of 'problem dogs'. This almost universally entails the reinterpretation of all such anthropomorphic terms and assumptions in a more realistic light, including so-called dominant and submissive postures. It is arguably more dangerous, during practical interactions with dogs, to assume 'submission' than to imagine a dog is using aggression to 'dominate'. If we assume submission and that a dog is thus giving permission to be handled as we see fit, we do so at our peril (see Chapter 2, 'Dos and don'ts of behaviourally aware general practice').

ART AND 'DANGEROUS' DOGS

In his book *Dog – A Dog's Life in Art and Literature*, Iain Zaczek refers to the dog portrayed in the well-known mosaic in Pompeii. The mosaic depicts a tethered dog crouching and one can imagine barking. The mosaic has been named historically 'Cave Canem' and is therefore probably the earliest known 'Beware of the dog' sign. The author goes on to state that 'As well as offering companionship, dogs showed their goodwill towards humans by guarding their homes' and that this practice 'dates back to ancient times.' Damned if they do and damned if they don't, like the witch on the ducking stool, nothing could be a clearer or more accurate picture of the double bind today's dogs find themselves in. With little or no understanding of what makes dogs tick, this hypocritical and downright schizophrenic attitude towards dogs has been enshrined in legislation (see Chapter 11, 'Dangerous Dogs Act').

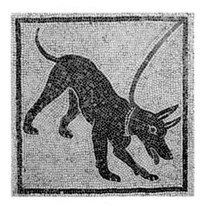

BREED CREATION

Very late on in the history of the domestic dog came the creation of official breeds, in other words, dogs which began to be selected for appearance and conformation only. The UK Kennel Club was formed in 1873 when a consistent set of rules and standards were laid down to describe how and to what criteria dogs should be bred in order to maintain a uniform size and appearance. A *Stud Book* was compiled the following year detailing the pedigrees of dogs known to have competed at various shows since 1859. Dog fighting having been banned in 1835, along with bear and bull baiting, dog shows provided an alternative form of sport whereby prizes could be won based on a judge's preference for an appearance rather than ferocity. Dogs were already being selected and bred from to enhance particular characteristics. The breed standards laid down what these characteristics should be.

Historically, conformation was inextricably linked to the particular function for which dogs had been both naturally and artificially selected for thousands of years and already a variety of anatomical shapes and sizes existed to be selected from. The seven breed groups currently listed by the UK Kennel club loosely reflect the dogs' original function. Selecting for function alone resulted in anatomical change. Among the most obvious examples are that, in selecting for running ability, long legs were produced, whereas any dog that was useful in negotiating a rabbit warren tended to have short ones. Other less obvious changes have occurred which have contributed to the function historically required. It has been recently established that there is a correlation between retinal cell distribution and nose length (McGreevy 2004). Dogs with long noses have retinal cells arranged in a streak rather than a spot and thus have extremely good long-sighted vision which is also movement sensitive. Hence the renowned ability of the Greyhound and variants thereof to see no point in running anywhere unless there's something seemingly alive to chase and to live as supreme examples of the couch potato the rest of the time. The corollary is that short-nosed dogs have retinal spots, are relatively short-sighted and see the world rather more as we do.

Very recent research (Hecht et al. 2019) has shown that the neuroanatomy of the brain varies significantly according to the specific behaviour traits breeds have been selected for. Moreover, these anatomical changes persist even if the behaviours themselves are not being actively performed, as in dogs kept simply as pets and not required to work.

Despite the Kennel Club breed groups being based upon their historic function, whether a particular present-day dog could physically fulfil this function is highly debatable. Appearance and human taste is the sole yardstick by which breeds have been and still are deemed desirable and, in certain cases, seems to have produced anatomy far removed from the norm. Most brachycephalic breeds (having a shortened and overly broad skull) are of concern, suffering as they do with chondrodystrophy (a genetic skeletal trait affecting the development of cartilage growth plates). It is generally characterised by a normal sized trunk and shorter than normal limbs. Other associated abnormalities include lower jaws that protrude further than normal together with short upper jaws and crooked teeth, bowed front legs, and a crooked spine. This has resulted in a multitude of physical defects in breeds such as the Dachshund, Bulldog, Corgi, Pug, French Bulldog and Bassett Hound and is related to selection for a particular and apparently extremely popular appearance.

The removal of form so far from function has resulted in dogs so disabled and anatomically deformed that they can hardly breathe or walk, let alone run. Many require extensive surgical intervention to correct, or at least ameliorate, such inbred defects, a need which has led to the development of further veterinary expertise and, dare I say, opportunity. It is extremely worrying that it is now considered the norm for breeds such as the English Bulldog to be unable to give birth naturally and those chosen to breed from, and thus perpetuate deformities, must undergo elective caesarean sections in order to be able to reproduce at all. Indeed, certain members of the dog-related fraternity seem to have lost any idea what normal is.

This vicious circle of events has been aided and abetted by the selective advantage brought to dogs by paedomorphic (child-like) characteristics, such as large eyes and short noses (Waller et al. 2013). But this has been taken to highly detrimental extremes. Warnings to the public to 'stop and think before buying flat-faced dogs' seems at present to be falling on deaf ears as the French Bulldog returns to the top of the rankings as the UK's most popular breed, according to Kennel Club registrations in 2020.

Nor is the anatomy of long-nosed dogs immune to deleterious fashion whims. The German Shepherd, once an able working breed, has changed in profile from having a healthy horizontal back to one so sloping as to give shortened rear limbs, a crouched hind limb stance and unstable gait. A dog so affected, yet which won 'best of breed' at Crufts in 2016, caused a public outcry and led to a Kennel Club revision of the breed standard to include what some may say should be blindingly obvious, that a dog must be 'capable of standing comfortably and calmly, freely and unsupported in any way' (www.thekennelclub.org.uk/pressreleases).

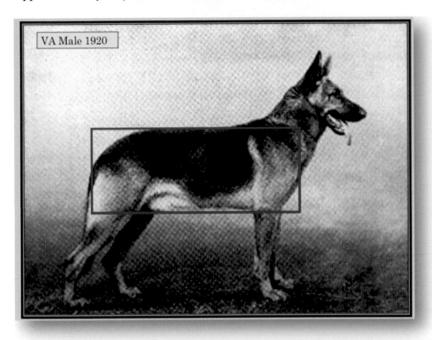

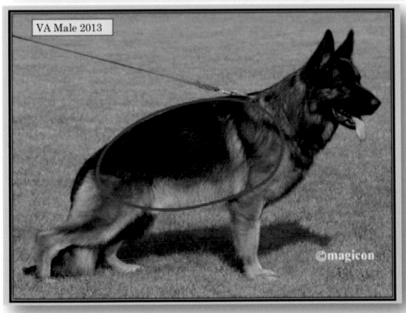

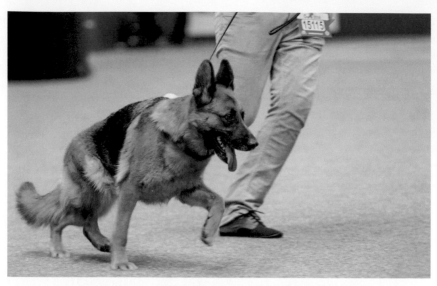

From an article by Henry Bodkin, *Daily Telegraph*, 28th July 2017.

The behaviour of the breed has also come under scrutiny after a Royal Veterinary College survey indicated that aggression, more prevalent in males, was over-represented as a reason for euthanasia requests (O'Neill, D. 2017). Whether such aggression was purely behavioural or related to pain caused by other significant defects was not clarified. During a visit to a military dog training centre some years ago, I was informed that all rescue German Shepherds, considered suitable for adoption and use as working dogs, routinely had their hips screened for hip dysplasia, owing to its high incidence. But suitability for working on one hand and reason for relinquishment on the other, was based upon readily displayed aggression. As a trainer there stated, 'These dogs already have the aggression. Now all they need is training.' Were these dogs thought 'unsuitable' for life as a family dog yet 'suitable' for military work suffering from underlying pain?

Although surgery is carried out of necessity on welfare grounds when presented with an individual animal, what of veterinary care and responsibility for the health and welfare of a breed as a whole? How can a society purporting to care so much for 'man's best friend' have allowed itself to become complicit in such a warped sequence of events?

The need and ability of people, particularly females, to nurture is demonstrated in all pet-keeping societies, and it is suggested that 'the ability to care for young animals was selected for, as an honest indicator of future quality as a mother' (Bradshaw 2010). Archaeological evidence for care-giving, not only of a young dog but a sick puppy, has been suggested by recent analysis of the contents of a 14,000-year-old human grave found near Bonn, Germany, among which was found the skeleton of a young dog of 28–29 weeks old. The dog appeared to have been well cared for, particularly as its teeth showed evidence of enamel damage typically associated with canine distemper infection, specifically between the ages of 19 and 23 weeks. As mortality is high, it is argued that the dog's survival must have relied upon intensive care and the attention reserved for those with whom humans had a strong emotional bond (Janssens et al. 2018).

Among five recognised social support systems, emotional support, social integration, esteem and practical support are all means whereby one's feeling of self-worth is *gained from* the altruistic and approving behaviour of others. The fifth, having opportunities for nurture, protection and the sense of being needed or depended on by others is generated by *giving to* others. It is further suggested that all of these roles may be fulfilled by dogs, including the fact that caring for them as dependants can bring satisfaction and social approbation (Serpell 2002). The fact that the company of a dog can improve one's self-esteem is even acknowledged in popular cartoons and greetings cards. Concern for animal welfare itself may stem from the adaptive nature of care-giving. The more we care, the more we seem to need to care, and care-giving becomes a goal and occupation in itself.

Paradoxically, therefore, in providing a sense of being essential to a dog's survival and welfare, not only is dog rescue considered a worthy cause engendering a certain social kudos but may have led to the, possibly unwitting, creation of needy dogs. But the 'caring, nurturing' trait has seriously backfired if it has brought with it the positive selection for frank deformities in dogs which subsequently need inordinate amounts of care in order to satisfy human need for canine company and emotional necessity.

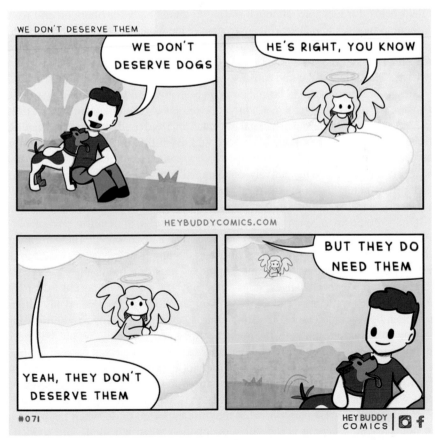

Reproduced with permission from Hey Buddy Comics.

It has been suggested that alterations in appearance may also have resulted in dogs less able to use visual signals effectively and so be misunderstood by other dogs. Protruding eyes in the front of the face may appear to be staring, interpreted as threat, particularly if there is only a deformed remnant of a tail with which to clarify intent.

I myself was once persuaded to enter a pet food manufacturer's 'Rescue Dog of the Year' competition with my German Shepherd, who had been suffering with severely neglected and infected demodectic mange (to the extent of almost complete baldness) and with acute symptoms of social deprivation when I took him on at the age of 5 months. He made a complete physical recovery, though some mental 'scars' remained. We came in third place. At the time, it seemed a great way to highlight the cause of animal welfare. In hindsight, to publicise dog food by competing on the grounds of whose pet had suffered the most, and whose 'rescuer' had done the best job, seems questionable at best.

Breed-specific behaviour is well recognised, demonstrated *par excellence* in the trainability and sheep-herding abilities of the Border Collie. What might be thought of as symptoms of an 'obsessive-compulsive' disorder in other breeds, these traits are actively encouraged when useful and have resulted in the Border Collie being the dog of choice when competing in agility. The same traits are not so convenient if displayed out of context, when chasing cyclists or attempting to herd children by nipping at their heels, for example, although staring at tennis balls for hours on end waiting for them to move is tolerated with amusement. One wonders however, how much the behavioural reputation that breeds carry with them (and which may be enshrined in their breed standard) creates an expectation in owners that they have a need to behave this way. Thus, the 'shake and kill' for example, in terriers is excused as normal.

Owners are encouraged to keep their dogs both physically and mentally stimulated to ensure the dog's needs are met. Physical exercise is recommended several times a day and when at home much mental stimulation is advised to combat behavioural problems by keeping the canine brain occupied. By fulfilling a perceived behavioural need, and even accentuating it, are traits which are ill-advised, potentially problematic and even dangerous being actively encouraged? In addition, the dependency that results from attending to every 'need' and treating dogs as 'family' may result in over-dependence, with separation distress becoming a worrying welfare concern.

It may come as a surprise to learn of the results of studies carried out on free-ranging street dogs ('streeties') such as that carried out in Bangalore, India (Pangal 2019), regarding how dogs choose to occupy themselves when left to their own devices and without human interference. The study found that, regardless of season-related weather changes, dogs spent 45% of a 24-hour period asleep, 32% lying still just 'watching' and 23% 'moving'. 'Moving' comprised all activities other than being completely still – from simply scratching, eating and eliminating to walking, running and playing. It might be imagined that dogs would be chasing, fighting, stealing and generally making a nuisance of themselves for a much higher percentage of the time. But these dogs did not choose for themselves very much activity at all and certainly not the highly structured life that is often imposed upon them when under human control. Not only that, but for the typical household pet there is a huge contrast between what they are expected to do when people are, or are not, present. Sleeping is the safest occupation when left alone and sudden activity is expected when reunited. There is no gradual and relaxed change from one state to another and little opportunity for simply 'watching the world go by' (www.livesofstreeties.com).

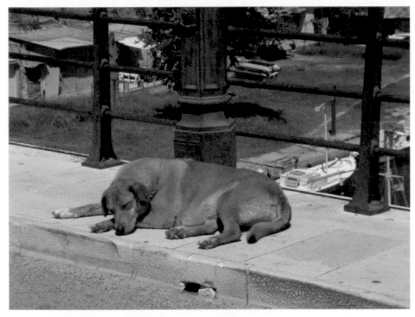

Dog in Corfu Town.

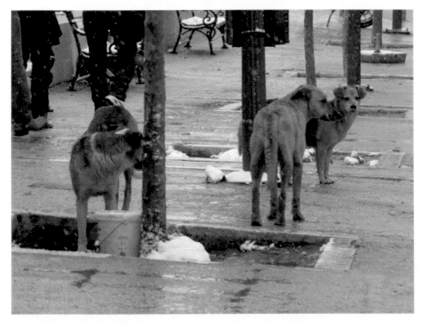

Street dogs in Athens.

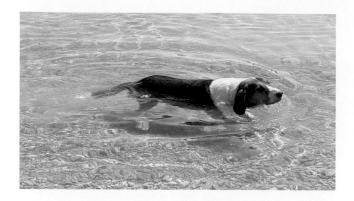

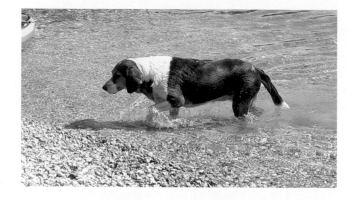

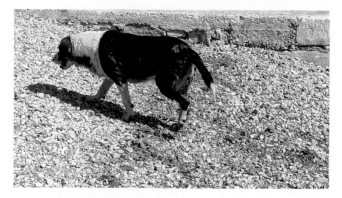

Swimming in Horto, Pelion.

And what is the effect of the artificial selection that now routinely exists when human society in its wisdom chooses which dogs should be allowed to reproduce and which individuals come to a genetic dead end? Are we reducing the 'healthy' gene pool by being 'responsible' and neutering all cross-breeds and mongrels of excellent temperament while allowing breed representatives based on appearance only to remain entire? In some ways, the current vogue for 'designer cross-breeds' is a good thing, in that the genes available upon which selection can act is increased. But only if all aspects of a truly healthy dog, both physically and behaviourally, are recognised. Prospective dog owners must be made thoroughly aware of the disasters that may arise if they are influenced solely by the foibles of fashion.

Deliberate selection for behavioural traits which would be of advantage to all breeds in the modern world seems non-existent apart from when human need is paramount. This is demonstrated most clearly when assistance dogs are both chosen and purpose-bred for their non-reactive, tolerant and 'biddable' nature. But rarely is the combination of behavioural attributes that would make up the 'ideal pet dog' even considered. Selecting for dogs able to fulfil the often conflicting vagaries of human need should be paramount. Above all, selecting for the ability to remain content when 'home alone', while ensuring at the same time that activity is not overly encouraged when owners are present, would do much to pre-empt re-lationship breakdown.

SUMMARY

1. The domestic dog is not a pack animal and has no concept of dominance and submission.
2. It has retained ancestral communicative gestures designed to maintain harmony in a social animal.
3. These gestures have proved highly adaptive to the species as a whole, despite anthropomorphic misinterpretation.
4. Canine aggression is a normal response when appeasement fails and has been lauded in certain contexts and condemned in others.
5. Artificial selection for fashionable appearance has created grotesque distortions of normal anatomy, which are contrary to the health and welfare of many dogs

CONCLUSION

The modern-day dog fits in with human society as best it can when attempting to meet our ambiguous, and often conflicting, demands. In many ways, it seems that they understand us better than we do them. It may be that the evolutionary goalposts are now moving too quickly for people, let alone dogs, to keep up. But if we are going to maintain the same uniquely close relationship with dogs into the future that has been developed in the past, we do owe them our full reciprocal understanding – what makes them tick, why we love them and how we, albeit hitherto unwittingly, bring out both the best and worst in them. Such understanding, if instilled from childhood onwards, will produce better informed adults in the future in all walks of life, to mutual health and welfare benefit everywhere.

2 Dos and don'ts of behaviourally aware general practice

> **This chapter covers**
> Promoting behavioural health
> The concept of behavioural husbandry
> What to do and not do to prevent/minimise behavioural damage

I am fully prepared to admit that my first interest in dog behaviour was sparked purely out of self-interest and being wholeheartedly fed up with dogs who 'misbehaved' in my consulting room. As I had somehow gained the reputation of 'being good with dogs', I may well have been unwittingly landed with more than my fair share of patients who were likely to bite me.

A practice where I worked (before my behavioural epiphany and before computerisation – yes *that* long ago!) had written client record cards which were brought into the consulting room by the client themselves. To warn the attending vet of a patient's propensity for violence, yet supposedly keep the information hidden from the client, the code 'DOS' was inscribed on the top right-hand corner of the card. It did not of course require the brain of Einstein to work out that this was 'SOD' written backwards. But this is how such dogs were routinely viewed and treated: vicious creatures who had to be manhandled and 'dominated' in the only way they understood so that we could get our job done. During this time, I became adept at fashioning makeshift muzzles out of a roll of bandage and using a dog catch pole to extricate such 'sods' out of their kennels. I even remember myself saying, when about to do something I knew a dog was likely to object to, that *'nice* dogs wouldn't mind a muzzle, and *nasty* dogs needed one'. I cringe at the thought of how I justified my ignorance.

And what was a 'sod'? With the wisdom of hindsight, simply a terrified animal who had learned to bite first and ask questions later.

While working in a subsequent practice, I was more often found walking a dog round the block to demonstrate the advantages of a head collar. I had found the judicious use of bits of food combined with a head collar far preferable to a choke chain to control a dog. Creating a backlog of my clients in the waiting room and irritating the receptionists was the only price to pay. But not all practices were so accommodating.

I once did one day a week for a local one-man practice. I had already become aware of how important it was to try to ensure that every dog, particularly young ones, enjoyed as many aspects of a surgery visit as possible. To this end, I habitually put a tub of tasty dog 'treats' next to the stethoscope (before they became fashionable to wear round the neck!), thermometer and other essential consulting room paraphernalia. The practice nurse followed my lead and began to dole out dog biscuits in the waiting room.

I took great satisfaction when clients remarked how much happier their puppy was for its second vaccination than the first. But I of course could not be aware of how they had felt when my employer administered the second injection, after I had given the first. Nor did I realise that there were to be repercussions.

The unintended consequences of my actions therefore only became apparent when I began to notice that, every week when I arrived for work, the tub of dog treats had been deliberately put away by my employer at the very back of the furthest cupboard. This was the way he tacitly expressed his thorough disapproval.

We parted company shortly thereafter.

So why do we as vets and other veterinary professionals need to worry about anything other than treating physical ailments to the best of our ability?

An American Veterinary Medical Association mission statement regarding the human-animal bond reads, 'The veterinary surgeon's role in the human-animal bond is to maximise the potential of this relationship between people and animals'.

With this in mind, I first introduced the concept of **behavioural husbandry** in an article I wrote for the *Veterinary Record* sister publication *In Practice* in 2007.

The aims of behavioural husbandry were two-fold:

- To create an appropriate management system by giving guidance at start of a dog-human relationship. Opportunities can be created at the time of puppy vaccinations and during puppy parties and classes. The veterinary consulting room and surgery should be presented as a role model for the rest of a dog's life.
- To sustain the dog-human relationship by identifying and optimising the continuing management system. This includes the communication system between dog and owner, the relationship between dog and environment and awareness of the impact of veterinary intervention upon both.

I quote from the article:

Any form of veterinary intervention should at the very least, aim for limitation of behavioural damage and at best ('best practice') should achieve an improvement in the relationship between the dog and veterinary clinic and between the dog and its owner and/or its environment. (p. 541)

To fulfil this aim and implicit obligations, as well as enhancing the welfare of both parties, it is impossible to ignore the emotional and behavioural aspects of these relationships in favour of purely physiological illness and disease. In addition, rather than only addressing defects in the dog-human relationship which have already occurred – the client complains about destruction in the home, urinating indoors or being snappy towards the children, for example – the onus is now on all of us to be rather more proactive in our approach.

We must also realise that a relationship does not exist merely between a particular pet and its family, but between that animal and all the humans it may happen to come into contact with elsewhere, including those inhabiting veterinary surgeries. The dog which becomes progressively more hard to handle in the surgery over time, although frequently labelled as 'aggressive', 'difficult' or downright 'nasty', is in reality simply one whose behavioural needs and emotional welfare have been inadvertently damaged in the process of maintaining physical health or attending to physical disease.

On the other hand, an animal who is genuinely pleased to come to the surgery and whose behaviour and emotions have been nurtured in the same way as its physical needs is a tribute to the attending veterinary surgeon as well as its owner.

Here follows a summary of essential 'dos and don'ts' with brief explanations as to why and how they should be carried out or not, as the case may be. For more in-depth explanation where necessary, the more avid reader will be pointed towards elsewhere in this book.

DO ENSURE THAT COMPETENT BEHAVIOURAL 'FIRST AID' IS AVAILABLE IN-HOUSE

Much can be done to assist in cases of apparent behavioural 'emergency'. Emergencies often involve dogs which have just bitten for the first time. Without doubt, this will have caused considerable upset all round. There may even be a 'knee-jerk' request for euthanasia, as the myth of 'once a dog has tasted blood' is seemingly alive and well in the minds of some owners and, dare I say, veterinary surgeons. Offering to hospitalise the offending dog overnight to allow emotions to settle is a sensible first move. After all, the presentation may be as life threatening as a road traffic injury. Information regarding the incident can then be more rationally ascertained and analysed later.

If the in-house source of behaviour advice is an experienced veterinary nurse, ensure that by passing the client on to them, dealing with behavioural issues is not relegated to the realms of lesser procedures, such as suture removal or dressing changes. The importance of behavioural problems, particularly aggression, must be seen to be taken very seriously, even though an attending veterinary surgeon may have less knowledge in this regard than a veterinary nurse.

DO INCLUDE SOCIAL DETAILS ON THE DOG'S RECORDS AS A MATTER OF ROUTINE

Whereas companion dogs and other animals may be automatically listed on a client's records, other details pertinent to behavioural history may not be. These include the type of accommodation a dog lives in and whether it has a garden, how many adults and children are in the family and who goes out to work and who has more time to spend at home. It is most important to ascertain if the dog has attended training classes and what training methods have been used (see Chapter 3 'Peri-operative behaviour counselling').

DO APPRECIATE EVERY DOG THAT BEHAVES WELL IN THE PRACTICE AND REWARD ACCORDINGLY

Wherever a dog happens to be, if it is behaving in a way that is not causing annoyance, the chances are that the appreciation of 'lack of bad' behaviour will not be expressed to the dog in any meaningful way. In fact, if it is not misbehaving, it may not even be noticed at all. Rarely do we watch a dog anywhere and try to work out why it is not barking, not pulling on lead, not lunging at passing cars and not jumping up at passers-by. All our attention is drawn towards those dogs displaying less-than-desirable habits (see 'Human attention as a reinforcer' Chapter 4). Yet understanding and promoting good behaviour is equally if not more important than analysis and treatment of the 'bad'.

It follows that ….

DO NOT TAKE GOOD BEHAVIOUR FOR GRANTED

This is possibly the biggest mistake we can ever make. I am at the risk of repeating myself here but this is so important – wherever a dog is in the practice, ensure dogs behaving well are noticed and appreciated. Dogs are deemed to need controlling when they positively do things we do not approve of. Rarely do we ensure that a reward is given simply for doing nothing, when just standing still and not reacting in any way may be the most convenient thing to be doing. 'Good' behaviour, (i.e., not annoying or dangerous but appropriate for the context) must be acknowledged and our appreciation demonstrated to the dog meaningfully. If we do not, then the result may well be erosion of the 'good' in favour of behaviours which gain the most human attention. In this way, we risk the deterioration of behaviour over time. A client's observation that 'he used to be fine when he was younger' is evidence that the state of 'being fine' had never been remarked upon or rewarded and had been completely taken for granted.

However, further analysis of what 'being fine' actually entailed, specifically regarding what a dog's body gestures looked like when young, can be very revealing. The more subtle signs of stress and threat-aversion, such as nose licking and crouching down with laid-back ears, may already have been present but not interpreted for what they were. The puppy may have been attempting to divert unwelcome attention by wriggling and even appearing 'playful', the 'faff-about' mode of dealing with stress (see 'The Ladder of Aggression' Chapter 5). It is therefore likely that appeasing and threat-averting behaviour was indeed present but, from the dog's perspective, did not result in the expected polite response. Rather than achieving the socially acceptable 'back off for a minute please', efforts to control the young dog increased, leading to devaluation of these subtle signs.

DO PRAISE THE BEHAVIOUR, NOT THE DOG

The phrase 'Good boy' is universally used as praise and is therefore thought to reward the dog by making us pleased. This assumption is based on the possibly misplaced belief that dogs' *raison d'être* is purely to bring us pleasure. It follows therefore that achieving this goal of creating human pleasure will alone be sufficient to reward a behaviour. Whereas our pleasure will indeed be rewarding if contrasted with crossness, 'good boy' as used in training class or at home more often comes to signify 'at ease'. The phrase is uttered after the dog has obeyed us or at the end of a training task such as a 'sit stay' or 'stay down'. It will therefore have come to mean 'do what you like now' and is more accurately described as a 'release' command. It is far more effective to repeat 'good sit' or 'good stay' to keep a dog doing what you want it to. Human pleasure or praise is thereby linked precisely to the behaviour you want to continue. Say 'good boy' as often as you like after you've successfully looked into the ears, taken the blood sample, clipped the nails or given an injection.

DO OFFER EVERY DOG SOME FOOD AS IT ENTERS THE CONSULTING ROOM

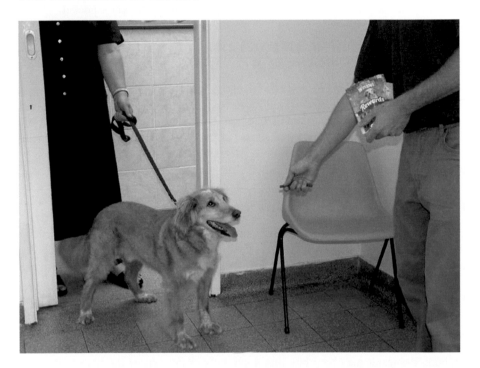

Offering food as the dog enters acts is a rough guide to its emotional state. The dog's response can be very informative and will immediately assist in giving an idea of how a dog may behave as the consultation progresses. Food is an **unconditioned reinforcer.** As such, a dog doesn't need to learn that food is necessary and good and very rewarding to eat! If the dog turns his nose up, it does not mean he is not hungry or that food has become unimportant. Instead, in the context of the consulting room, eating has gone way down on his list of priorities. He may be simply looking for an escape route or possibly gearing up to bite. It all depends on how the interactions between him and the environment, of which you and the owner are part, progress.

DO NOT ALLOW ANY DOG TO BE DRAGGED INTO THE CONSULTING ROOM

If at all possible, even small dogs which could be picked up easily, should be allowed to walk in of their own accord. For anxious animals, trying to stay outside rather than entering is the obvious choice for them. It's up to us to alter that choice – not by coercion, thereby reducing a dog's behavioural options, but by increasing their options. To achieve this, ask the owner to enter first and encourage the dog to follow, not necessarily by using food as an inducement (as already mentioned, dogs in this emotional state may not be able to eat) but because the owner appears to be abandoning them. The dog is simply more likely to follow the owner to keep their company. This effect is enhanced if veterinary staff stay behind the dog and owner as they enter. The consulting room is thus made to appear the safest, rather than most dangerous, option. The relief at catching up with the owner may well enable eating of the food already on the floor or appearing from the vet's pocket.

DO NOT IMMEDIATELY LIFT ANY DOG ONTO THE CONSULTING ROOM TABLE

Whatever the size of patient, instruct clients to leave the dog on the floor to begin with. Allow some exploration of the room first, instructing owners to let the lead trail. Exercise an obedience command, such as to sit, before the dog is lifted up. Size of dog and the impossibility of getting some onto an examination table should not be the only determining factor in the decision. Many smaller dogs will also be happier on the floor.

DO REMEMBER 'TRIGGER STACKING'

This catchy phrase has latterly been coined to describe the way that events a dog finds hard to deal with may stack up on top of each other until only one, maybe relatively insignificant, event is sufficient to tip the emotional balance and provoke aggression. Entering your consulting room may well be the final straw in terms of your patient's tolerance. In addition to stimuli immediately present, all that has been previously experienced that day will affect the emotions of the patient as well as be 'remembered' by the dog's physiological stress response. If prior or concurrent negative experiences and their physiological and emotional effect are not taken into account, the result may be a bite that apparently 'came out of the blue'.

We may be unaware of, or forget in the heat of the moment, how long it takes for the physiological stress response to return to normal and that if another stressful event occurs *before* this has happened, then the response to the second event is heightened. Thus, individual events the dog may cope with without showing outward signs of stress or anxiety at all accumulate until a critical mass is reached. Jean Donaldson in *The Culture Clash* (1996) explains that all dogs have a 'bite threshold' which can be reached if sufficient successive stressors, or triggers, are experienced. Although a prior 'growl threshold' is also illustrated, in some dogs there may be no growl before a bite or it may be so imperceptible or momentary as to more or less coincide with a bite. Other dogs may have been ill-advisedly punished for growling. As an increase in threat is the absolute opposite of a growl's purpose, such dog will therefore have learned to dispense with this valuable warning sign as having no use.

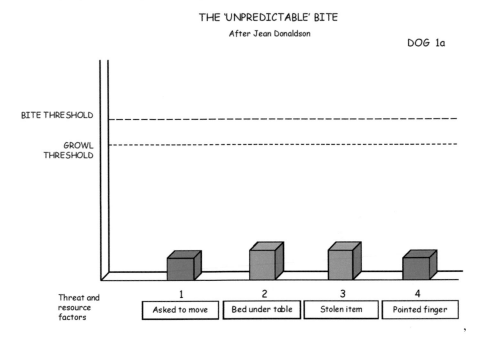

THE 'UNPREDICTABLE' BITE

After Jean Donaldson

DOG 1a

BITE THRESHOLD

GROWL THRESHOLD

Threat and resource factors

1	2	3	4
Asked to move	Bed under table	Stolen item	Pointed finger

,

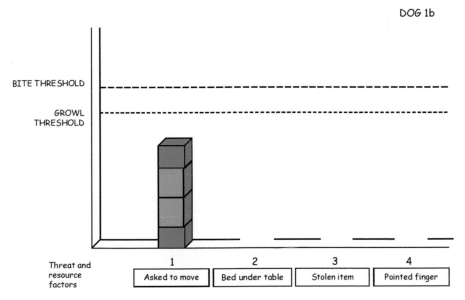

DOG 1b

BITE THRESHOLD

GROWL THRESHOLD

Threat and resource factors

1	2	3	4
Asked to move	Bed under table	Stolen item	Pointed finger

THE 'UNPREDICTABLE' BITE

After Jean Donaldson

DOG 2a

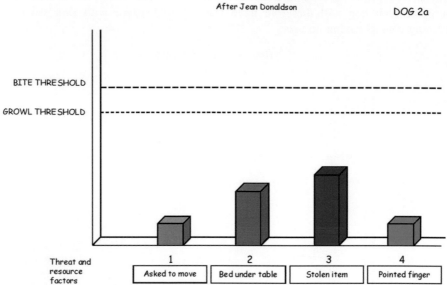

BITE THRESHOLD

GROWL THRESHOLD

| Threat and resource factors | 1 | 2 | 3 | 4 |
| | Asked to move | Bed under table | Stolen item | Pointed finger |

THE 'UNPREDICTABLE' BITE   '

DOG 2b

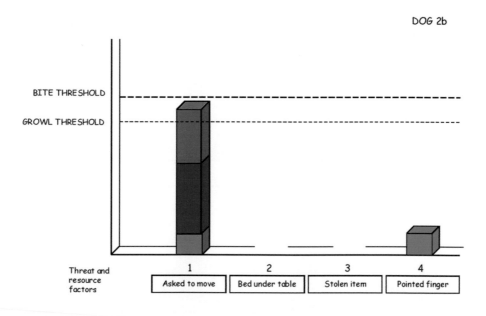

BITE THRESHOLD

GROWL THRESHOLD

| Threat and resource factors | 1 | 2 | 3 | 4 |
| | Asked to move | Bed under table | Stolen item | Pointed finger |

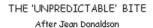

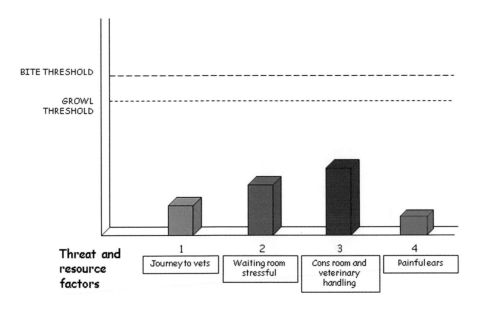

THE 'UNPREDICTABLE' BITE

After Jean Donaldson

Dog 3a

BITE THRESHOLD

GROWL
THRESHOLD

**Threat and
resource
factors**

1	2	3	4
Journey to vets	Waiting room stressful	Cons room and veterinary handling	Painful ears

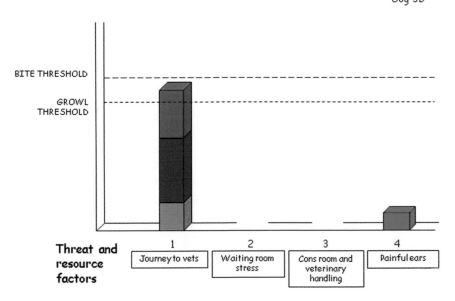

Dog 3b

BITE THRESHOLD

GROWL
THRESHOLD

**Threat and
resource
factors**

1	2	3	4
Journey to vets	Waiting room stress	Cons room and veterinary handling	Painful ears

Stressful events which may have occurred before a dog enters the consulting room may include having had an 'argument' with another dog during a walk earlier in the day or having the experience of the car turning right at a roundabout, thus predicting 'vets' rather than left towards the park and encountering a busy waiting room containing other stressed animals. Being lifted onto the consulting room table and lastly, the sight of a stethoscope or syringe are the 'last straws'. It becomes easy to see that there is nothing sudden in the mind of the dog who 'suddenly' snaps.

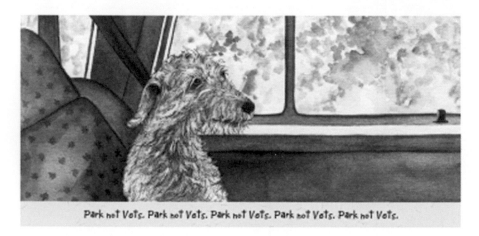

Park not Vots. Park not Vots. Park not Vots. Park not Vots. Park not Vots.

Reproduced with permission from Team Little Dog.

DO USE KNOWN 'OBEDIENCE COMMANDS' AS CHANGERS OF EMOTION AS WELL AS BEHAVIOUR

All thoroughly taught and readily obeyed commands, regardless of training method, have a rewarding consequence (see Chapter 4 'What is obedience?'). There is a positive emotional change upon hearing, and in turn complying with, the command. This can be used to advantage in the consulting room and can help create an animal that is in a more positive frame of mind. A dog may view a food titbit very differently depending whose hand it's in – the owner's (always good news) or yours (ambivalent at best). The following diagram shows how food and a known command can be used to alter both behaviour and underlying emotion to the advantage of all.

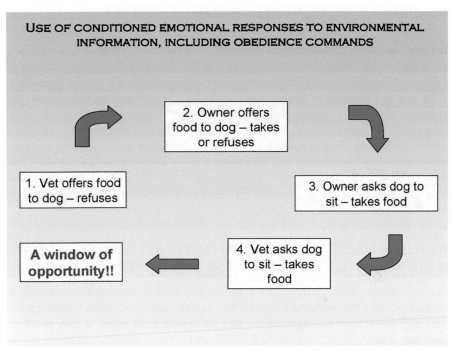

USE OF CONDITIONED EMOTIONAL RESPONSES TO ENVIRONMENTAL INFORMATION, INCLUDING OBEDIENCE COMMANDS

2. Owner offers food to dog – takes or refuses

1. Vet offers food to dog – refuses

3. Owner asks dog to sit – takes food

A window of opportunity!!

4. Vet asks dog to sit – takes food

© Kendal Shepherd 2008

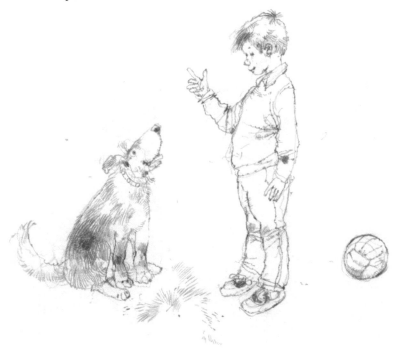

Illustration by Victor Ambrus.

DO NOT ALLOW VOICES TO BECOME RAISED IN THE CONSULTING ROOM

Dogs are, possibly uniquely, alert to the human voice and its tone and nuances. The sound of the voice conveys meaning and the tone may be very significant in its implications for the dog, depending on past experience. So often the reaction of the patient to general chatter goes unnoticed by both attending veterinary surgeon and client. Discussion regarding possible diagnoses, treatments, prognosis and, last but not least, the cost of it all, may become animated and even emotional. Setting aside the implications of tone of voice and emotional content, the impact of decibels alone in a reverberant room can have an untoward effect upon a patient.

Be aware of the dog's responses at all times, however subtle, and keep voices as quiet, calm and unalarming as possible.

DO NOT MUZZLE ANY DOG WITH IMPUNITY, SIMPLY IN THE KNOWLEDGE THAT IT CANNOT BITE YOU

All precautions should be taken to avoid behavioural damage whether a dog is muzzled or not. Once wearing a muzzle has become associated with fear and pain, overt aggression may be triggered by **any environmental event which predicts muzzling**. This could be the sight of a needle and syringe, the concern in the owner regarding how their dog will behave or even the fact it was raining during the last vet visit. This was brought home to me all too clearly when I was informed by the owner of an outwardly calm German Shepherd, brought in for vaccination, that 'you'll have to muzzle him'. No sooner had I made the first move by simply reaching out towards the drawer in which the muzzles were kept than the dog transformed into a lunging, snarling 'savage'.

An alternative to muzzling is accustoming a dog at home to a head collar with muzzling action and for it to be put in place before the dog enters. The jaws can then be gently held shut and the head controlled without the need for muzzle placement and the associated alarm it may cause.

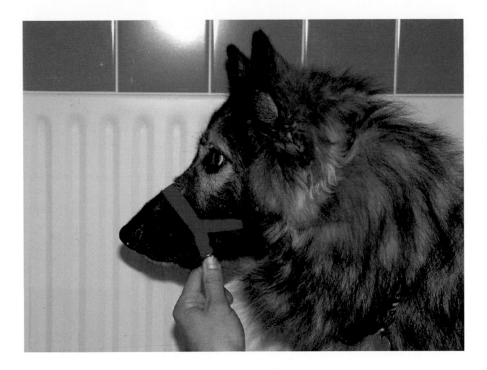

DO CARRY OUT THE LEAST PLEASANT PROCEDURE LAST OF ALL AND, IF POSSIBLE, AT AN EXIT POINT

The pressure of time one feels under in any consultation may create the temptation to get any potentially stressful procedures over and done with as soon as possible. Far better is to spend time as described above to create a more amenable frame of mind in one's patient *before* proceeding to give a potentially painful injection. If carried out as close to the way out of the consulting room as possible, uppermost in a dog's mind will be his imminent departure. A dog trapped in the furthest corner away from the door will feel far less hopeful.

DO CONSIDER EXAMINING ANXIOUS AND FEARFUL DOGS OUTSIDE THE PREMISES

Many dogs will be better behaved in the car park simply because many of the cues which predict veterinary handling and therefore trigger fear and anxiety are absent. Giving such a dog more freedom may, seemingly paradoxically, result in better behaviour than if enclosed in a small room. The dog will be in a calmer emotional state and is likely to be more amenable to handling.

DO NOT EVER INTERPRET A DOG GOING 'BELLY UP' TO YOU DURING EXAMINATION AS 'SUBMITTING' TO YOUR ATTENTIONS!

Last but by no means least, this is another extremely dangerous mistake to make. In reality, one could be not only a whisker away from being bitten but also well on the way to convincing the patient that, next time, he'll go straight to more obvious ways of repelling you and without warning. However many books you may have read persuading you successfully that this how wolves, and therefore their descendants, domestic dogs, are supposed to demonstrate their subservience, nothing could be further from the truth. Often labelled 'passive' as opposed to 'active' submission, and therefore seemingly less dangerous, a 'belly up' dog is at its most vulnerable. It has already given up on appeasing 'actively' by laying ears back, raising a paw, crouching and tucking the tail under. What else can a dog do to express its discomfort?

This is, however, an ambivalent signal and must be interpreted in context. A dog may well go belly up with his owner, who is known and (hopefully) trusted, and this gesture may be interpreted by owners, and used by their dog, as an invitation for a tummy tickle. But this may not be true even for all members of a family and their visitors, let alone in the veterinary context. The safest interpretation to make is always that the dog wants to be left alone. This is exactly how a well-socialised adult dog will behave towards a belly-up puppy. A sniff or two at the head and inguinal region and the puppy is left alone. The young dog thereby becomes confident and secure in its ability to communicate. If manhandling were to follow instead, the exact opposite happens.

To demonstrate your understanding of the gesture, take a step or two back and allow or actively encourage the dog to stand before continuing your examination. The dog then has a choice, which of itself is less stressful.

By the same token, **never** force a puppy onto its back in order to demonstrate your 'dominance' and elicit supposed 'submission'. By so doing, you will devalue the young dog's inherent belief in this ultimate calming gesture and its social value when expressed voluntarily (see also Chapter 5 'The Ladder of Aggression').

CONCLUSION

Although this may seem a lengthy list of instructions, just one of any of the above will improve one's awareness of the mental state of canine patients and, in turn, their behavioural responses. Although avoiding the emergence of aggression is a major concern, this advice should be applied to all patients, not only those thought to need it. Ultimately their relationship with all things veterinary will change for the better. We must remind ourselves that it is not just the health of canine bones, skin, eyes, heart, liver and lungs that needs preserving. 'Bad' behaviour (including aggression) can be as big a threat to a dog's life as conventional illness. The fundamental relationship between dogs and their owners, and in turn human society, is of equal importance. This cannot be achieved unless the behaviour of dogs is considered in every aspect of veterinary care.

The veterinary surgeon's role in the human-animal bond is to maximise the potential of this relationship between people and animals.

3 'Do as I do'

For the most part during a consultation, we give advice on what clients should do to care for their pet. This may be regarding general routine care, such as diet, grooming and worming, or more specifically about the condition being treated at the time, such as bathing an abscess or redressing a wound, how many times a day tablets need to be administered or when they need to come back for a check-up. We do this without necessarily demonstrating exactly what they should do every step of the way– although personally I always gave a demonstration of how to apply ear ointment.

Following manufacturers' instructions to count the number of drops to dispense, I found, was worse than useless. It guaranteed that in order to ensure the correct number of drops, the nozzle had to be outside the ear. The said ointment got nowhere near the vertical and horizontal canals where it needed to be and was more likely to be found spattered all over kitchen cupboards after vigorous head shaking. Hence there resulted many apparently intractable cases of otitis externa, a particular beef of mine.

Interestingly, the advertisement accompanying the recent launch of a single-dose topical treatment for otitis externa for application during consultation only cites 'solving the owner compliance challenge' as a distinct advantage of this new preparation. It also states that 'it's easy to underestimate how challenging owners find treating their dog at home. Even the most well meaning, committed owners may struggle but won't necessarily admit this to their vet'. In other words, have small animal vets ever been fully cognisant of the difficulties both owner and pet face at home?

In any vet-client relationship, there are concomitant expectations. The expectation of the vet is that the clients should do as they have been told, and of the client that they must try to follow their vets' instructions to the letter. (Would that it were true, do I hear you mutter?)

These assumptions cannot be made when it comes to the handling of a pet dog. The word 'handling' might even be better replaced with 'communication with' their pet. 'Handling' means just what it says on the tin – the dog must have some form of 'hands on' restraint in order to get a particular job done. Communication, on the other hand, is so much more important. It implies that owners must inform the patient of what they are about to do and what the dog is expected to tolerate during examination in order to prepare the dog in advance for what is about to happen. A dog is far better able to cope with events when there is already a known strategy in place as to what to do. So often, even the sight of a bottle of ear drops triggers a rapid departure from the room. It is therefore incumbent on the attending veterinary surgeon to ensure that whatever a dog's chosen coping strategy happens to be, it is convenient for the vet and comfortable for the patient.

What bodily position will be better for the dog to adopt – standing, sitting or lying down? Which part of the body needs to be touched? What result has the dog been led to expect when having a paw lifted or ear touched? One can talk about correctly applying the principles of learning and what pressures can be brought to bear to ensure a dog complies with requirements until one is proverbially blue in the face. But nothing is more valuable than actually showing, by your own practical approach, how to do it. Not a word need necessarily be spoken, or the word 'behaviour' even mentioned: simply 'do as I do' demonstration is enough.

This is not just for one's own satisfaction in successfully completing a consultation without a struggle and without further frightening a recalcitrant patient. It will also have far-reaching effects on how the dog is dealt with in the wider world. While clients may not do as they are told, they are susceptible to copying what they have seen. This is particularly true of children. If they observe a parent shouting at or dragging a dog off the forbidden sofa, this is how they may try to it themselves, thereby creating a serious risk of being bitten. The same is true for veterinary surgeons as role models. If the vet forcibly restrains a dog, or alternatively asks a couple of nurses in to do it for them, this may be deemed acceptable and to be emulated by the client.

How much better therefore to show how a dog can learn to tolerate veterinary attention by gaining something the animal wants, or alternatively being rid of what it does not want, as a direct result of such tolerance?

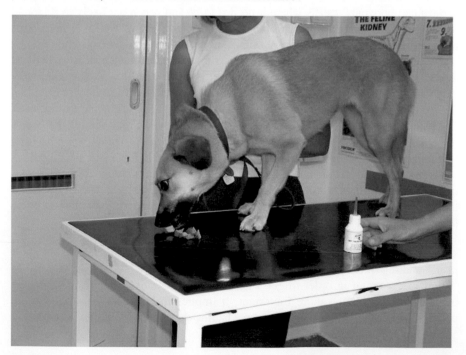

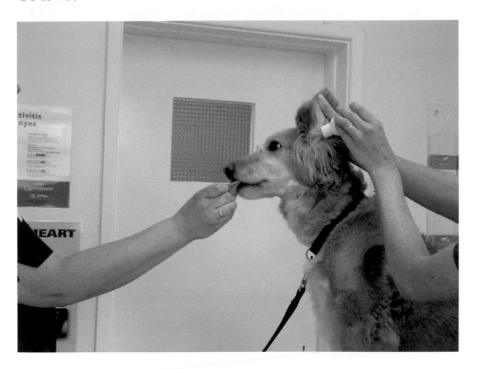

FROM PUPPY CLASS TO CONSULTING ROOM

First of all, what a puppy learns in a 'party' or class must extend beyond the remit of the veterinary nurse or trainer and enter into every aspect of the veterinary premises, including most importantly the consulting room. If puppies were 'fine' in class but not so fine once they've reached their first birthday, then the lessons taught early on have not been sufficiently rehearsed in all the contexts in which a dog is expected to succeed. Particular attention must be paid to those behaviours which best allow veterinary handling and examination, namely, the sit, the stand, the down and the roll-over. Although taught as obedience exercises in class and possibly in a client's sitting-room, they are generally very ill-rehearsed, if at all, in the veterinary consulting room. It is therefore imperative that vets are also involved in the puppy training process, if only out of a sense of self-preservation. For a particular behaviour to be deemed worth doing, then there must always be both anticipated and tangible rewarding payback for the dog, wherever the puppy happens to be. There is little point in giving a food treat for an obedient sit in a puppy party only for a sit in the consulting room to result in a painful injection. A young dog's newly formed trust in veterinary aspects of the world can thus be completely demolished.

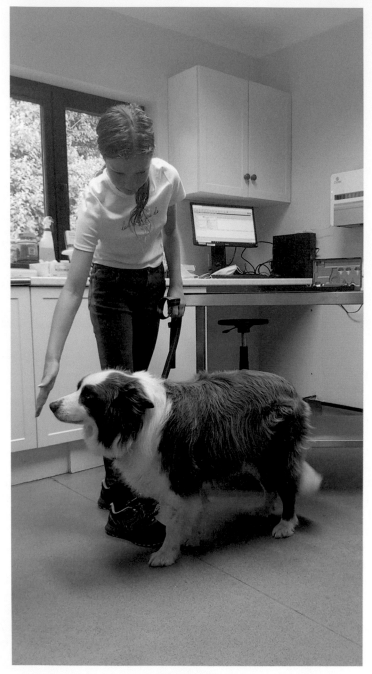

The 'stand'.

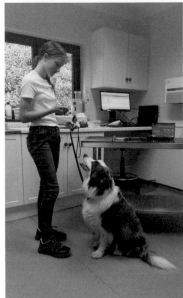

(a) The 'sit'.

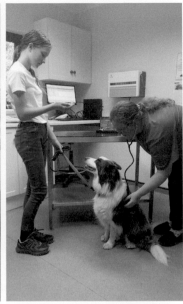

(b) The 'sit' for examination.

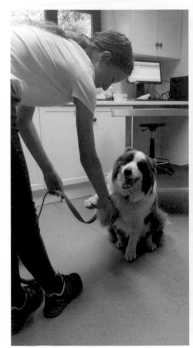

(c) The 'give' paw.

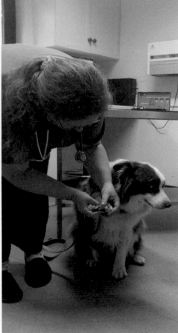

(d) The 'give paw'
for examination.

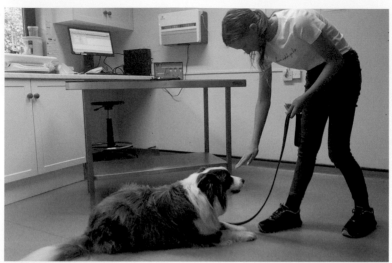

(e) The 'down'.

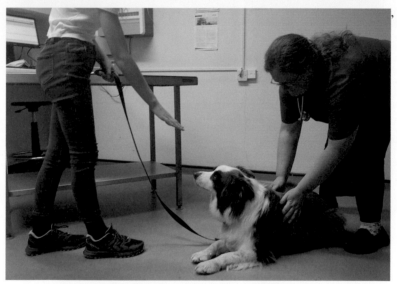

(f) The 'down' for examination.

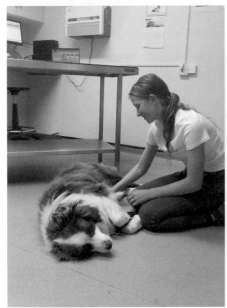
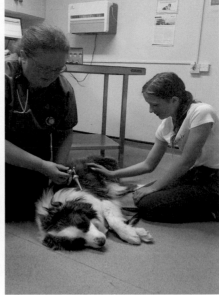

(g) The 'lie down/roll over'.　　　　　(h) The 'lie down/roll over'
　　　　　　　　　　　　　　　　　　　for examination.

THE PUPPY VACCINATION

The young puppy's first visit to the surgery is the most crucial and attitude forming that it will ever experience. It is essential that this visit is made as pleasant and as educational as possible, however long it takes. Lessons learned now may be remembered for the rest of the dog's life – for better or for worse. If handled well, the adult dog may forgive a multitude of sins as previous pleasant memories help protect against future unpleasant-ness. If handled badly, a dog readily prepared to bite when threatened is created, at any time in the future and in any similar context. The majority of the available consultation time should be spent ensuring that the puppy not only enjoys himself but begins to learn the behaviours that will be the most convenient all round for the rest of his life. There are very few puppies who will not eat in the consulting room at this stage in their veterinary careers if tasty food is both offered 'for free' and given as rewards for suitable behaviour. It is essential that this is carried out before anything unpleasant has happened to them. Trying to 'make friends' after the puppy has been made upset is far harder to do and may be impossible. Do not therefore be misled into thinking 'let's get the nasty stuff over and done with as quickly as possible'. Extra time spent now is an investment in your re-lationship with the growing dog which will reap huge dividends in years to come.

It is arguable that discussions regarding worming, diet and neutering should be left to a competent veterinary nurse while the veterinary surgeon's time is better spent teaching the puppy to sit on the consulting room table, using food as a lure. By contrast, the most important lesson a puppy must not learn is that being held firmly predicts pain and discomfort. I firmly believe that it is the accompanying enforced restraint which adult dogs come to object to rather than the injection itself. To avoid this unfortunate association being made, the moment the injection is given, the puppy must be let go and allowed to eat offered food. Evidence of success are smiling owners and a puppy who sits willingly on the table when presented for his second vaccination.

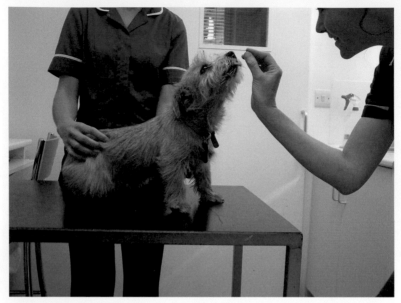

Reinforce 'sit' on consulting room table with food.

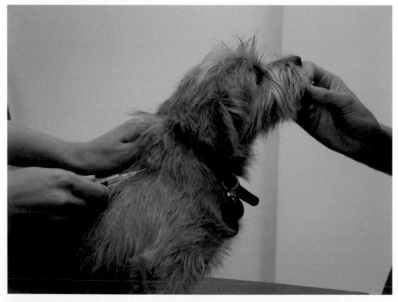

Hands off and give food at same time as injection administered.

POSITIVE VERSUS NEGATIVE REINFORCEMENT

We must not imagine for a minute that positive reward in the form of goodies is the only way to provide a rewarding experience in the consulting room for a dog. Indeed, a dog may not feel like eating at all in this context. The relief at the removal of an unpleasantness (i.e., potentially you!) as a 'negative reward' can be very real and a potent emotional bargaining tool. As far as possible, therefore, the behaviours a dog should ideally learn are only those which facilitate veterinary examination while at the same time also work best at getting unwelcome veterinary attention to retreat. Whatever behaviour seems to result in a vet backing off will be the one that is reinforced and chosen next time. Being asked to sit to earn the relief of leaving the consulting room may reinforce the behaviour better than any food, however tasty.

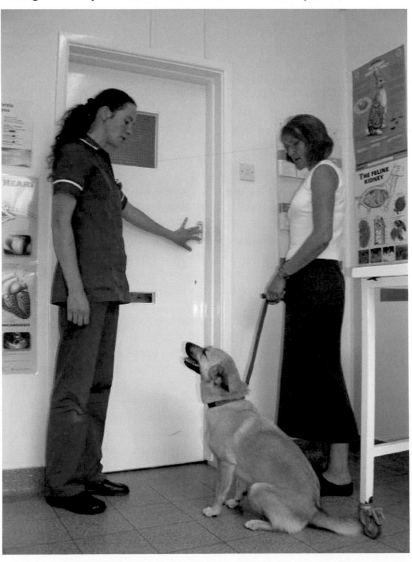

Biting, growling, wriggling or sitting still are all feasible options to get rid of our ministrations as far as the dog is concerned. The choice of which to reward and reinforce is up to us. If from puppyhood, only calm behaviours are selected and rewarded, whether by positive or negative means, then these behaviours will remain high up in a dog's repertoire throughout its life, even in a veterinary context.

CONDITIONED EMOTIONAL RESPONSES

Although a dog may not take food if offered from the hand of a veterinary surgeon or veterinary nurse, the same food item may be readily accepted from the hand of the owner. The explanation is simply that one hand has fewer negative connotations than the other. For a certain number of dogs, however, they are simply too worried by the environment of the clinic to take food even from the hand of the owner. But if the same dog is asked to sit by the owner (at the same time ensuring that the owner's body language looks as if they are relaxed and happy rather than stressed by being in the surgery) a considerable proportion of dogs will not only comply with the command but will then also accept the food item. Why?

Previous experience of the word 'sit', the body language of the owner and anticipated reward has produced a **conditioned emotional response**. Whenever this familiar word is heard and congruent gestures seen, an associated emotional change for the better occurs. This allows the dog to relax sufficiently to feel like eating. In other words, the sit command itself results in eating rather than a dog sitting to be given food. It is then highly likely that a sit command issued by the veterinary surgeon or veterinary nurse will also be obeyed and food eaten as a result. Once this breakthrough in communication is made, a window of opportunity is created whereby a dog's view of the surgery and consulting room can be improved (see 'Conditioned Emotional Responses' diagram in Chapter 2).

LABELLING OF BODY PARTS

The more predictable the results of a particular context are, the more secure a dog will feel in how to cope with it. Consistent words for particular body parts can become associated in a positive way with, for example, handling of 'ear', 'paw', 'neck', 'tail' and 'back'. This process can be very usefully demonstrated in the consulting room and advised to be thoroughly rehearsed at home. At the same time as reaching forward towards the body part, a food reward should be offered and the body part named. The food is then given as contact with the body is made. The clicker can be employed to specifically mark a body part and to predict a rewarding result for tolerance of touch (see Chapter 4 'Clicker training').

Simple touch should progress to actual handling, for example, massaging and squeezing the skin overlying the neck, inserting a finger into the ear and looking at individual toes, all the while rewarding the dog for tolerance. Two people can be involved in this exercise at home as well as to demonstrate the process in the surgery, when the owner can be instructed to supply the food (with or without a 'click') to coincide with a vet or nurse reaching to touch and handle whichever body part is being labelled. Which person utters the word can vary, as can who does the touching and the offering of food. In this way, a predictable and pleasant outcome is created for the dog regardless of who is involved.

This exercise should ideally be carried out *before* the said body part is in pain; otherwise, it will then be much harder to replace already existing negative associations with positive ones.

PERI-OPERATIVE BEHAVIOUR COUNSELLING

I attended a CPD day some years ago on cruciate surgery. There were several mentions of how difficult aggressive, boisterous and disobedient dogs were to manage post-operatively and how this can substantially alter prognosis for the worse. I began to wonder about behaviour counselling specifically in preparation for the rigours of surgery, confinement, prolonged lead walking, hydrotherapy, etc., within a specialist referral situation. It seemed a natural extension of the field of behaviour therapy, both in prevention and treatment of problems. Although the concept was inspired by the threatened waste of a specialist's work and the welfare implications for the dog, the issues involved are equally relevant to general practice.

It seems that there are foreseeable defects in the relationship between dog and client which may compromise the success of surgical and medical intervention. Although this applies to animals treated in both general and referral practice, in view of the standard of excellence that referral centres otherwise provide, it may be that there should be an increased duty to provide the necessary behavioural care to ensure medical and surgical success. A first step is to become aware of the need for such care from both human and canine perspectives.

Of necessity, the advocacy of peri-operative counselling involves making certain predictive assumptions about the behaviour of both patient and client, how they interact together and how surgical and medical prognoses may be affected. These presumptions can be confirmed or corrected by asking questions prior to surgery. Gathering information routinely regarding a patient's home life and habits for clinic records has already been advised (see Chapter 2) but questions particularly pertinent to the peri-operative period are shown in the following box.

How has your dog been trained?
(*What emotional responses have been conditioned and why?*)
What cues (words/gestures) is he familiar with?
(*Use the same ones after admission*)
Are there any concerns regarding reactivity to noises?
(*Protect dog in hospital/early intervention for treatment indicated*)
Where does dog usually eliminate? On command or 'asks' to go out?
(*Gravel/grass/earth/concrete*)
What is the dog's reaction to other dogs?
(*May govern kennelling choice*)
What is usual lead restraint? How do they behave on lead?
(*Pre-prepare with head collar for less coercive control*)
How does dog react to grooming – at home or at the groomers?
(*If better behaved at groomers, consider owner-absent examination. Basket muzzle training if needed*)

I realise that such preventative advice is entirely in opposition to the diagnostic approach to behaviour that has been presented to the general practitioner in the past. It has been made to seem mandatory for a specific problem to be identified before treatment can commence. In other words, there has to be a diagnosable problem from which the dog is suffering with definable causes and specific treatments. But I would argue that there is a common approach which can be taken in both prevention and treatment of all behaviour 'problems'. The environmental changes that the dog perceives as a result of medical intervention are no different to any other context a dog may experience, and the dog will respond, for better or worse, according to the same rules.

At the risk of repeating myself, the advantages are many from everybody's point of view.

FROM THE VETERINARY SURGEON'S PERSPECTIVE

- The ability to handle the patient in the surgery is intrinsic to thorough clinical examination, investigative procedures, diagnosis and treatment. Conversely, the 'difficult dog' may preclude appropriate treatment. How amenably the patient behaves in the surgery is therefore crucial.
- Post-operative requirements may include multiple veterinary check-ups, the wearing of protective collars, medication (oral or topical), confinement at home, prolonged lead exercise, redressing, etc. Unwillingness or inability of the owner or patient to comply with such advice may compromise recovery.
- Fear and pain-associated aggression may worsen with successive veterinary treatments, however minor.
- It is far easier to have good relationship with a client if their dog behaves appropriately. Not only will the attending veterinary surgeon be able to

concentrate on the job in hand rather than whether they will get bitten, the vet will simply be perceived as kinder and more caring if handling the dog in question does not involve brute force and several nurses.

FROM THE OWNER'S PERSPECTIVE

- Much post-operative advice entails manipulating a dog in a way an owner may never have contemplated or attempted. Advice such as lead exercise only for six weeks will not be complied with if the dog is uncomfortable or impossible to walk on a lead. Oral medication or topical application of, for example, eye drops will not be carried out if to do so carries a risk of physical harm.
- Unaccustomed and enforced confinement highlights problems such as destructiveness and house soiling.
- Unaccustomed and enforced handling may induce threat-based aggression.
- Most obedience training is class or exercise based, rather than home based. If a dog is apparently well behaved at home, commands such as the 'sit-stay' and 'watch me', which would be extremely useful to enable a dressing change or eye drop application, may never have been practised *in situ*. An owner may feel suddenly bereft of means of communication indoors and surprised at their apparently 'disobedient' dog.
- Non-acceptance by the dog of imposed restrictions will be viewed as 'bad' behaviour and may either be condoned or be met with the human default value of punishment. Both are deleterious to the dog-human relationship.

FROM THE DOG'S PERSPECTIVE

- The post-operative period is likely to involve radical alteration to a dog's normal routine. Few dogs have been trained or habituated to post-operative requirements.
- For most dogs, obedience training (i.e., the communication of owner requirements) is exercise based. Enforced restriction or absence of exercise and confinement at home may result in a dog with no effective guidance.
- Veterinary intervention is one of the biggest tests of canine temperament and tolerance. Many dogs are at best merely tolerating veterinary procedures of all kinds.
- Although initially fear and pain based, aggression becomes a learned strategy to avoid handling and restraint in subsequent similar situations.
- Owner anxiety and the necessary extra care given during illness or surgery and recovery is at risk of becoming a habit. Worse than usual behaviour may be excused and condoned on the basis of 'feeling poorly'. Dogs have no way of knowing that they themselves are ill or injured, only that the parameters of daily life have inexplicably changed. A dog may no longer be expected to 'come here' or 'sit' when asked, for example. Owners may not be aware of this change and, even if they are, they themselves realise it is only temporary.

The change in owner behaviour, even for a relatively short period of time, may however lead to permanent expectation of change on the part of the dog. Subsequent demands for obedience may be viewed as unexpected challenges and result in conflict.

From the perspective of all, predicting what changes will be needed, and making appropriate behavioural alterations *before* they're needed post-operatively, will be highly beneficial.

The stress of veterinary intervention therefore highlights defects in a dog's education and relationship with its owners. This may result in simply the increase in significance of irritating, attention-seeking habits and deterioration of behaviour generally or to the more serious emergence of aggression. Owners may be entirely unaware, and indeed have no need to become aware, of such defects in routine day-to-day life, when an illusion of obedience is created by the normally unstressed and apparently 'well-behaved' dog. Home-based mental exercise may need to replace physical exercise in preparation for the restriction of the post-operative period and be used to establish meaningful dog-owner communication.

SUMMARY

1. As attending veterinary surgeon or nurse, every procedure performed should be considered as a demonstration of how the client should ideally continue at home.
2. There is no such thing as a 'quick puppy vaccination'! This could be the most crucial learning experience of a dog's life and should be allocated the time it deserves.
3. Incorporate puppy class lessons into the consulting room and elsewhere in the practice building.
4. Consider the importance of negative as well as positive reinforcement in guiding a dog's behaviour.
5. Consider peri-operative behaviour counselling for any procedure, but particularly in preparation for elective surgery.
6. **Encourage colleagues to 'do as you do'!**

4 What is obedience?

The client and I stood in the consulting room – she trying unsuccessfully to restrain her excited Springer Spaniel and me, equally unsuccessfully, attempting to examine him. This was in the days before I understood that such behaviour on the part of the patient was the 'faff-about' response to threat and stress, whereby he was seeking to repel unwanted attention by wriggling vigorously. Unbeknownst to me at the time, had I and his owner persisted in forceful and coercive handling, the dog may well have been left with no other option than to snap and bite.

As it was, I simply labelled him a 'badly-behaved' dog who was wasting my time and stretching patience to the limit.

The owner, sensing my tacit disapproval, retaliated, 'He's a highly clicker trained show dog, you know!'

By this stage in my behavioural career, I was aware of what 'the clicker' was and how it was supposed to function, but I resisted the temptation to ask why it had been left at home if this had been the primary means whereby the dog was accustomed to being given information. But it was the revelation that he was a show dog which proved most helpful. I knew that, having attended ring craft classes, a solid 'stand-stay' was a prerequisite for the show ring and being examined by judges. By the same token, I was told that a 'sit' was a complete 'no-no', as the last thing a show dog should do was park his bottom the minute a judge's hands got anywhere near the rump.

The 'stand' command was duly given by the owner and understood by the dog to mean 'Let this stranger run their hands over you without moving'. Lo and behold, the dog obeyed. From then on, the examination proceeded smoothly and I was able to commend the client on how well the dog was trained. However, one could almost imagine the dog himself raising eyes to Heaven at the stupidity of mankind and asking, 'Why on earth didn't you just say what you wanted me to do in the first place?'

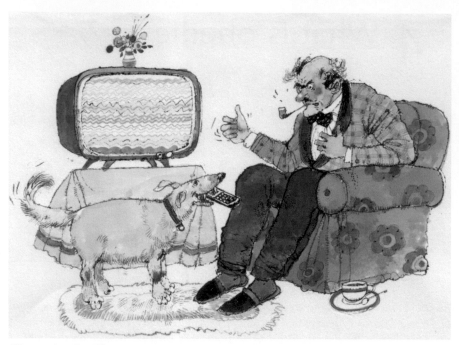

Illustration by Victor Ambrus.

Many valuable lessons were learned during this potentially disastrous encounter which really focused my mind upon the true nature of obedience and how easily we can confuse dogs by our actions and clumsy communication. Dogs after all are responding to, or ignoring, environmental events all the time in whichever way they see fit. Why do we imagine that what we say and do are so special? And if a dog appears not to listen or understand, whose fault is it?

WHAT IS OBEDIENCE?

Standard definitions of the word 'obedience' are all along the lines of the following, readily provided by Google dictionary:

> compliance with an order, request, or law, or submission to another's authority

Others include the following:

- 'Willingness to obey orders' *Chambers Pocket Dictionary*
- 'Submission to another's will' *Oxford Dictionary and Usage*
- 'Complying with rules' *Penguin English Dictionary*
- 'Doing what you are told' *Oxford School Pocket Dictionary*

It is hardly surprising therefore that when asked to say what obedience is and to apply it to dogs, the average owner universally replies with utter confidence and no small a hint of 'what a stupid question!': 'It means he must do as he's told!' The implications of this, at best, oversimplification and, at worst, damaging mis- understanding are several and profound. They are the cause of much conflict and mismatch between human and canine expectations.

Dogs are first and foremost expected to know that there are rules and what those rules are. Obedience is equated with submission and they are expected to defer to an authority. They are expected to know what words mean. Obeying 'orders' implies the involvement of threat and coercion in carrying out the order. All these inter- pretations feed readily into the concept of dominance and hierarchy. Whether we are conscious of the fact or not, implicit in all the definitions is that an obedient individual would really rather be doing something else. In order to be obedient, therefore, they must lose out.

This inevitably brings dogs and people into conflict. For the health of the dog- human relationship in general, and when counselling individuals, it is always essential to thoroughly clarify exactly what we all mean by 'obedience' before attempting to tackle the problem at hand. It may even be that, once this is explained, owners can begin to answer their questions and to solve 'problems' for themselves.

My own definition is this:
An obedient dog is one whose own choice of behaviour can be successfully altered to coincide with that of the owner.

This definition emphasises both that the dog has a choice in the matter and that the owner must have determined in advance exactly what they want the dog to do in order to instil obedience. It does not, however, indicate *how* the dog's mind should be changed.

It is worth pointing out at this juncture that the owner is not the only source of information to which a dog may respond. Yet all too often, owners assume that they are all-important and that, in every circumstance, they should be the most important item on the dog's horizon. Broadly speaking, **obedience training** refers to in- formation and instruction emanating from the owner only, as usually happens in the standard training class. **Behaviour modification,** on the other hand, although in- evitably involving owner-centred training, acknowledges the effect that other fea- tures of the environment have on a dog. Such influences may inadvertently 'train' a dog as well, if not more efficiently, than any process applied deliberately. In be- haviour modification, environmental events as well as owner behaviour are ma- nipulated to effect behaviour change in the dog for the better.

Let's take a typical example of 'environmental training': the dog that continues to bark at passers-by despite their owner's efforts to stop him. A dog is not to know that 'passers-by' are going to pass by anyway without his intervention. Inevitably, when they do, his barking is rewarded by the potential intruder's retreat and its apparent success. Dogs may deliberately seek out and remain in the best 'look-out' position (often the back of the settee next to the window) in order to be 'successful' as often as possible.

ON WHAT BASIS DO DOGS CHOOSE BEHAVIOURS?

We are all familiar with the 'carrots and sticks' metaphor with respect to guiding behaviour, whether of donkey, dog or child, but are perhaps not as *au fait* as we should be with what forms each can take and why they 'work'. According to the definition above, the outcome of the application of carrot or stick ought to be the exact behaviour we want the dog to perform. This is straightaway at odds with what the average dog owner needs, which is simply to find a means of stopping the annoying stuff. The human default position with regards to altering any undesirable behaviour of fellow man or beast is always to try to prevent it, generally by some form of punishment. Behave or else! Sticks may appear to have instantly gratifying results, but do they teach the dog what to do instead of being annoying? If used indiscriminately, without forethought or understanding, they may seriously backfire.

What are the means whereby outcomes for a dog are created and, with a modicum of luck, learned? Reward for getting it right or punishment for getting it wrong? It comes as a sobering thought when pointed out that the dog training fraternity have over time been far more inventive when it comes to sticks than carrots. Choke chains, correction sprays (human and bark activated), electric shock collars and so-called 'Freedom Fences' (buried electric shock fences) are all intended to punish wrongdoing while the humble food reward for getting it right needed no lucrative reinvention.

It must also be taken into account what outcomes have a rewarding or punishing effect as far as the dog is concerned. We know what would be nice or nasty from our own perspective, but not necessarily from the dog's. A hug from the owner may be enjoyed, but not if a child or stranger tries to do the same thing. An owner's disapproval may be highly emotionally significant whereas that of a stranger simply viewed as a threat. The value and impact of rewards and punishments also vary according to context. How much does a dog want to gain a reward or avoid a punishment at any particular moment in time? In the consulting room, close contact with the owner may override food as a motivator and admonishments pale into significance compared to the desire to escape a vet's clutches.

A LITTLE BIT OF THEORY

REWARD AND PUNISHMENT

Reward is defined as 'the consequence of an action which renders that action **more likely** to be repeated'.

Punishment, on the other hand, is defined as 'the consequence of an action which renders that action **less likely** to be repeated'.

In addition, both rewards and punishments can be **positive** and **negative**. In **positive reward**, something desirable is **gained**. In **negative punishment**, something **desirable** is **lost**. In **positive punishment**, something **unpleasant** is **experienced**. In **negative reward**, the **unpleasant stuff stops**.

Clear as mud? Confused? This is not surprising especially when the sort of punishments we consider to fit the crime for fellow humans may be, technically speaking, nothing of the sort. A punishment can only be defined by **result**, that of a reduction in crime, *not* by how many weeks one spends behind bars or how big the fine is. Both these are negative punishments, as the perpetrator is deprived of freedom or money in order to teach him a lesson. Retributive, 'an eye for an eye' or 'tit-for-tat' behaviour is not punishment.

The nature of a punishment or reward can only be evaluated by the dog itself and its success or failure judged by the behavioural result.

It is frequently necessary to clarify this to owners – that it is only how a dog sees things that matters, not what we think should be significant. It may be assumed that punishment only occurs by physical means, by smacking for example, and that 'just shouting' cannot constitute proper punishment. Yet there is something that may have a far more potent effect on our canine companions than is generally realised: human attention. We must not underestimate the importance of how it is given or withdrawn, when it is given or withdrawn and for what reasons, and the consequent behavioural impact.

Dogs enjoy many things other than food which, in the right context, can be used to 'train' them. The supply or withholding of pleasant as well as unpleasant experiences can be used judiciously to strengthen behaviours we want and weaken those we don't. Of the essence is the word 'judicious'.

The problem is the confusion in people's minds, including those of trainers, as to what is really happening in the mind of the dog. It is easy for most people to understand that positive reward, for example in the form of a piece of hotdog, given to a dog for sitting when asked, will act as a reinforcer and increase the likelihood and frequency of sitting occurring. They may also grasp that they must withhold the said hotdog until the dog sits. But do they realise, that in doing so, they are negatively punishing all other behaviours, other than the sit, that the dog tries in the meantime? And that the withholding of a specific intended reward will only 'work' if accidental reward for the wrong thing is not coming from elsewhere in the meantime?

Even less well understood is the relationship between punishment and negative reward (or reinforcement). Is it more important for a positive punishment to stop a behaviour (sheep chasing for example) or for the behaviour which appears to cause the punishment to stop to be negatively reinforced? There is lack of appreciation of the role of negative reward in our routine daily interactions with dogs as well as when purposefully dealing with the extreme of sheep chasing. Yet if these principles are fully understood, it is easy to see how negative reward can be created in the mind of a dog out of almost every unpleasant experience. This is achieved, firstly, by being fully aware of what the dog will find unpleasant and, secondly, by deciding which behaviour the dog must perform to have the effect of stopping the unpleasantness, thus bringing the potent emotional reward of relief.

Great skill and understanding is required regarding how each pressure is brought to bear upon behaviour in order to use them deliberately and why manufactured punishing devices (including those utilising electric shock, ultrasonic sound and compressed gas) can be so easily abused. The accompanying graph illustrates the difference in use of the two pressures (punishment and negative reinforcement) using electric shock as an example.

Do not for one moment imagine that punishing devices are being advocated here. I can think of nothing worse than deliberately putting a dog in a context in which they are sure to misbehave and then using some potentially painful gadget around their neck to punish them when they do so. The very idea is abhorrent. But understanding these principles can be used to explain why lesser aversives, such as getting cross or smacking, which happen on a daily basis, may seem to be effective at the time. Yet if getting cross 'worked', why do dogs keep repeating behaviours which make us cross? Why do they not learn what they should do instead? This is what mystifies owners.

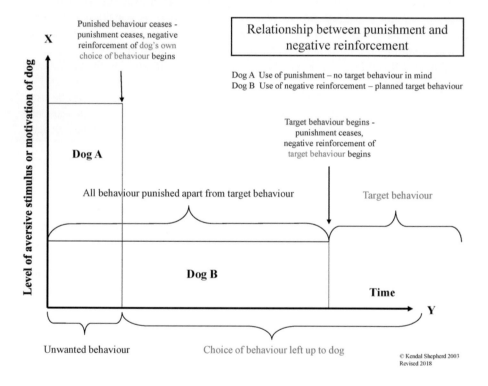

Dog A belongs to the average dog owner. All that the owner requires is for a particular behaviour (or several behaviours) to stop and stop as soon as possible. The dog is typically put in surroundings in which the behaviour occurs at its worst. The punishment is then applied at an intensity sufficient to interrupt the behaviour, at which point the punishment ceases. No thought is given to what the subsequent behaviour should be.

Dog B is in the hands of a skilled user of punishing devices. Rather than simply stopping a behaviour, a desired target behaviour is aimed for. The dog is put in the

least arousing situation to begin with and all behaviours other than the target behaviour are punished. As soon as the target behaviour is performed, the punishment
ceases. It is therefore rewarded by absence of the aversive.

For both dogs A and B, the motivation for the unwanted behaviour (or how much
the dog is 'driven' to do it) must be taken into account. **Dog A** is typically put in a
situation where the motivation is very high (the dog is already chasing sheep for
example). If the dog is just looking in their direction but not chasing them, there's
nothing to 'punish' yet, right? Wrong! By the time chasing has begun, the dog
will be so aroused that the intensity of punishment required to interrupt chasing
will be correspondingly very high. There is therefore a great risk of unacceptable
very painful levels of aversive being proportionally applied. Even so, the dog may
override pain in favour of chasing, resulting in multiple applications of shock.

Dog B may be just looking at sheep or walking slowly towards them. The intensity
of punishment required to 'change the dog's mind' will be correspondingly low but
will continue until the target behaviour is reached (turning to look at trainer for
example). The risk of failure and of inadvertently causing pain or distress is far lower.

Another way to explain the emotional effect of reward and punishment is to use
the accompanying Scale of Emotion diagram. This diagram describes (in much
simplified form) that all training methods work by producing positive emotional
change, whether in the form of relief at the avoidance of punishment (negative
reward) or satisfaction in gaining a resource (positive reward). It also emphasises
that all training is more effective if a dog is in emotional 'neutral' to begin with.

© Kendal Shepherd 2003

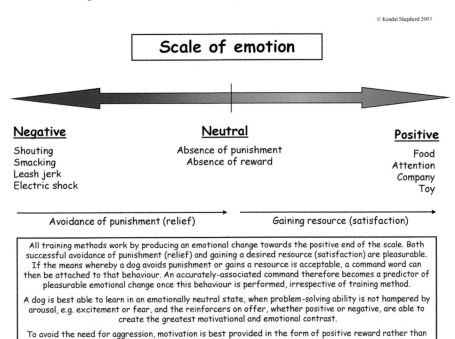

Scale of emotion

Negative
Shouting
Smacking
Leash jerk
Electric shock

Neutral
Absence of punishment
Absence of reward

Positive
Food
Attention
Company
Toy

Avoidance of punishment (relief)   Gaining resource (satisfaction)

All training methods work by producing an emotional change towards the positive end of the scale. Both
successful avoidance of punishment (relief) and gaining a desired resource (satisfaction) are pleasurable.
If the means whereby a dog avoids punishment or gains a resource is acceptable, a command word can
then be attached to that behaviour. An accurately-associated command therefore becomes a predictor of
pleasurable emotional change once this behaviour is performed, irrespective of training method.

A dog is best able to learn in an emotionally neutral state, when problem-solving ability is not hampered by
arousal, e.g. excitement or fear, and the reinforcers on offer, whether positive or negative, are able to
create the greatest motivational and emotional contrast.

To avoid the need for aggression, motivation is best provided in the form of positive reward rather than
avoidance of punishment, ie. emotional change from neutral to positive.

However much one disapproves of deliberate punishment in practise, we cannot deny the theory underpinning its proper use and that, if used knowledgeably with excellent timing, it can be effective. We also cannot deny that the human default value is to get angry, raise voices, threaten and smack and that being dealt with in this way is what domestication has led the dog to expect. Even so, we should not condone the deliberate application of potentially abusive techniques and devices. Rather we must understand the principles that govern their use, including the power of negative reinforcement, in order to explain to clients why the things they do instinctively when dogs misbehave may appear to work or may go disastrously wrong.

For all undesirable behaviours, there are three 'golden rules'.

1. We must have a clear idea of what we want the dog to do instead and thoroughly train that behaviour.
2. We must not put our dogs into such difficult situations that they misbehave and we feel forced to shout louder, jerk the lead harder or 'up the ante' on an electric shock collar remote control.
3. We must positively reward a dog when he gets it right, however long it takes and however angry they have made us feel.

In other words, an educational leaf could be taken out of the 'punishment' book and used to explain the principles that apply to all dog training and owner education. And, of course, if reward is offered before a dog becomes aroused, it will work just as well, or better, to guide behaviour in the appropriate direction, than a punishment applied after the event.

However we decide to train our dogs, they must be set up to succeed, not fail.

There is still much confusion, debate and frank sabre-rattling between certain 'old-school dominance-based' trainers and those who advocate 'reward-based' training only. Reward-based trainers are critical of old-school methods as unnecessary and potentially cruel just as the latter denounce the use of food as somehow 'spoiling' the dog. Semantics are manipulated deliberately to soften or harden the reality of effect on the dog concerned. 'Aversive' sounds nicer than 'punishment'. 'Tempting' or 'bribing' with food smacks of the criminal. Then there are the self-styled 'balanced' trainers who sit on the fence and jump down to one side or other as the need arises. But as with the wheel, we cannot reinvent or relabel what is going on to suit the impression we want to give.

Whereas police and military dog training used to epitomise the dominance and coercion-based approach, times are gradually changing. Positive dog training began in the Seattle Police Canine Unit by Steve White in the United States (www.proactivek9.com) and now been continued in the UK by police dog handler and trainer Guy Williams (www.positivepolicedogs.wordpress.com). Coming from a background of rehabilitating his own rescue dogs, he found that what he had learned in the past was completely at odds with what he was then being taught as a novice dog handler. Trying to introduce change has, however, met some considerable resistance. Might any change necessitate embarrassing corporate acknowledgement of previous mistakes based on the misunderstanding of dogs?

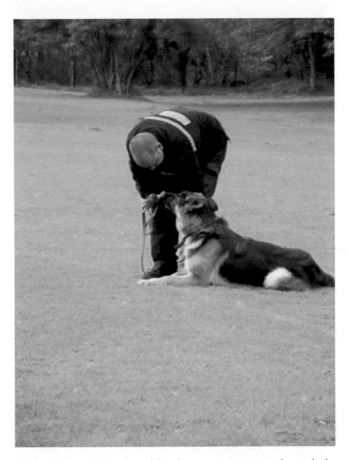

Dog put into 'down' position by pressure exerted on choke chain and with threatening hand gesture, body posture and tone of voice (positive punishment of anything other than the "down").

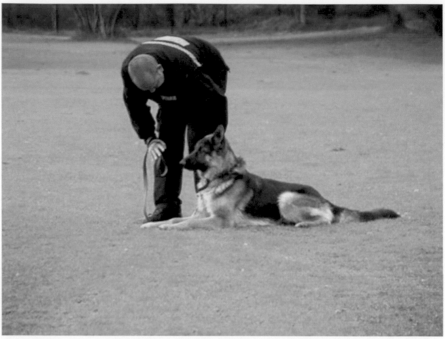

Once dog is in correct position, pressure on choke chain and physical threat ceases (negative reinforcement).

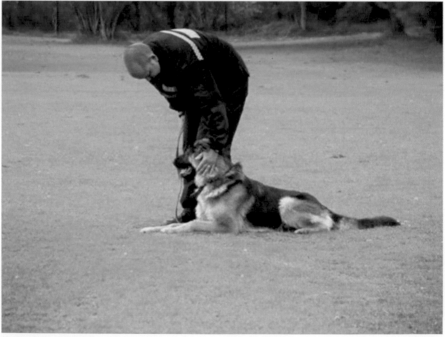

Dog then praised and petted (positive reinforcement).

The 'guru effect' I have to thank Dr. Myrna Milani for introducing me to this term years ago. It describes the inability of those who have set out their stall based on a particular premise to be open to new ideas and concepts. To do so causes cognitive dissonance and the perception that changing their mind might weaken their position as a 'guru'. Dog trainers are not immune to this effect. In this regard, I particularly applaud Victoria Stilwell who radically and publicly changed her approach from the dominance and hierarchy-based days of the television programme 'It's Me or the Dog' to her present enlightened stance.

MIXED MESSAGES

What happens when what we say is in conflict with what we look like and we thereby send incongruous and conflicting messages? Which of the two means of communication will have given the most evolutionary advantage to the dog? This will have come to be of overriding importance and is therefore paid the most attention by dogs in the modern day.

A dog is guided by the amalgam of what we look and sound like (incorporating facial expressions, bodily position, limb gestures and tone of voice). But of the two, what we look like is of overriding importance. Advanced training is required for dogs to respond accurately to words alone. As humans find it difficult to give instructions which are emotionally neutral and without an accompanying expression, it is easy to be misled into thinking a dog understands words alone.

The domestication process has resulted in an animal uniquely adapted to read and understand our facial expressions. Many studies have confirmed that dogs are guided by human gestures, particularly pointing, and look to us for visual information when faced with a problem they cannot solve on their own. It also has been crucial for them to be sensitive to our emotions as often expressed visually and by tone of voice. This understanding has allowed dogs to predict what various human expressions and actions mean and what relevance in terms of outcome they have for the individual canine.

It is known that dogs show 'left gaze bias', an ability it was thought that only primates, including of course humans, possess (Guo et al. 2009). Emotion is expressed primarily in this left side, the right side of the brain being responsible for the processing of the emotions. It has been crucial for the evident evolutionary success of dogs to read human emotion, heralding as it does the emotions of affection, love, pleasure, happiness, sadness and of course, anger. This phenomenon becomes more pronounced when anger is shown, indicating that of all the emotions, being able to read and respond appropriately to human anger has been of the greatest benefit.

Considering how important it is therefore for dogs to see our faces, I have often pondered the impact cultural vagaries, which dictate that part, or most, of the face should be covered, have had upon dogs. In turn, I wonder how the possible behavioural impact on dogs has affected the attitude such cultures may have towards the dog. Is it just a coincidence that a fear of dogs is more prevalent in those cultures where the face is often covered? Has the inability of dogs to read the emotions correctly resulted in a mutual and potentially dangerous distrust?

Obedience training harnesses all these abilities. It is relatively easy to 'train' certain actions as long as we are doing as well as saying what we mean. The 'stand', the 'sit', the 'give paw' and the 'lie down', for example, are all behaviours which are in the canine repertoire anyway. All we should be doing to achieve compliance is adding a cue, both visual and verbal, which means 'Do this (particular action) now and there will be a reliably good outcome for you'. Both the visual and verbal information must, however, be congruent.

A dog being told to 'Go to your bed!' as a reprimand while pointing bed-wards will generally have no trouble in interpreting our meaning and be thought to be being 'obedient' as they scuttle away. But what of the dog being called to 'Come here!' angrily and with a finger pointing down towards to the owner's feet? Will he decide that staying away is the more sensible and safe option and therefore be labelled 'disobedient'? Should the owner who complains, 'He just doesn't listen!' look more to their own behaviour than that of their dog?

For a dog to readily understand what is required, the command or cue must be given visually as well as verbally. Not many owners attend training class with baby buggy in one hand and handbag or shopping in the other and yet this is how they may present themselves at the surgery. Nor do they ask a dog to sit or lie down while they themselves are lying on a sofa in the training class. yet this is how a dog standing annoyingly in front of the television is 'commanded' at home. Moreover, a dog is expected to pick out a single meaningful word from the stream of inducements to 'behave' themselves, without being given a clue as to what to actually do to avoid human ire.

In class, where food is used to guide a dog's decision making, a raised hand containing a titbit generally accompanies the 'sit' command. The appearance of the raised hand therefore comes to predict the reward of food. Yet without food in the hand, it is almost universal that the hand changes in appearance, often to a pointing finger instead. The predictive rewarding value of the signal is lost. The result – an apparently stubborn and disobedient dog who 'knows what to do but just won't do it!'

By the same token, if a dog has been trained to sit coercively with a choke chain around the neck and a heavy hand on the rump, he may suddenly become 'disobedient' if off-lead and the means of applying coercion are absent.

Dogs are not alone in being fully aware of when a punishment can or cannot occur. How many drivers slam on the brakes when spotting a speed camera yet consider it safe to exceed the speed limit if there is no visual warning? Hence the increasing use of traps and hand-held guns to catch miscreants unawares. But drivers are also invited to attend educational 'speed workshops' where there is first of all commiseration regarding common reasons for speeding, then the potential result of their crime is impressed upon them and, most importantly, information is supplied as to how to avoid speeding in the first place. The (negative) reward for attending such a workshop is the avoidance of points on one's driving licence.

For dogs, being informed of how to avoid punishment rarely happens. If the means of punishment is immediately evident, they sensibly will avoid the punishment itself but not necessarily in the way we want. They are not generally given information in advance of exactly what they should do to avoid it in the first place. They are therefore not given the opportunity to choose for themselves an acceptable and rewarding behaviour to perform.

We must acknowledge how uniquely sensitive the average dog is to our displeasure or anger and how intrinsic this ability has been to their success. Dogs are universally described as 'loving to please us'. Is it perhaps more accurate to say they will do anything it takes to stop us being angry? And have we unwittingly made use of this in training them? Anyone who attempts to prevent this age-old and evolutionarily ratified means of disapproving of their pet will be on a hiding to nothing. Even St. Francis himself might have been hard pushed not to be a tad annoyed if he'd discovered his dinner 'in the dog'.

We will never prevent owners automatically saying, 'Oi!' or 'Don't you dare!' in an angry tone of voice to interrupt or pre-empt canine misdemeanour. But we can explain that, at the same time, dogs must be shown what they should do instead. We should also be clear in our own minds about where and when the rewarding event happens after such admonition. When 'Go to your bed!' is 'obeyed', the cross tone of voice and words cease, providing relief and a rewarding event for the dog.

To put this all in the veterinary context, it goes without saying that most dogs would prefer to be outside the consulting room rather than inside it. Letting a dog leave the room can therefore be used as 'carrot' which is then given as a negative reward for a behaviour convenient to all. The 'sit' is simple, understood by most dogs and readily performed if potential consequences are made clear. Putting a hand on the door handle (predicting the reward of escape), and at the same time requesting a 'sit', will shortly result in a dog who sits out of choice, as opposed to scratching the door to be let out (see Chapter 2).

This lesson can then very usefully be transferred to the homes of those dogs who 'scratch at the door' when they need a wee. This habit may have unintended consequences as what may seem a convenient behaviour in one context creates a problem in another. While this behaviour may be acceptable when the owner is at home, what can such dogs do when their owner is absent? The obvious thing is to wee indoors instead.

HUMAN ATTENTION AS A REWARD

Dogs are adept at gaining our attention in a great number of ways – some convenient and cute, and some downright irritating. They are often termed 'attention-seeking' behaviours as if any dog sets out to deliberately gain this reward by manipulating us. While there are some behaviours which have been selected for by humans as useful to alert us, such as barking in Ray Coppinger's 'doorbell dog' and raising a paw to 'point' in the gundog, many have simply been found to attract our attention and hence are more accurately termed 'attention-getting' behaviours. Only once a dog finds that certain behaviours do indeed gain our attention can they be adopted as truly attention seeking.

These behaviours are not always desirable ones, and the more disruptive or annoying a dog is, the more likely it may be that he is successful in gaining our attention. Owners must therefore be warned about how easy it is for annoying behaviour to become a habit, and the attention they give, with the intention of stopping a behaviour, has the opposite effect and prolongs it instead.

CROSS-CONTEXT LEARNING

Another lesson learned from my experience, related at the beginning of this chapter, was how important it is for dogs to be trained in all situations in which they are expected to know what to do. A dog may understand very well what is required of them when in training class or in the kitchen, but such learning does not automatically transfer to a different environment unless the dog has been trained **in that environment**. Children tend to understand that 2 + 2 = 4 wherever they are, but even small humans may find the answer to a simple sum tricky when concentrating on a game in the playground at lunchtime.

I was lucky with the simple show command 'stand' in the consulting room. Sufficient similarities between contexts existed for the Spaniel to make sense of the word. He was on a table, someone he was not familiar with was touching him and, above all, his owner, upon whom he relied for guidance, had shifted gear into 'show ring training' as opposed to 'being at the vets' mode. The traffic lights were working again.

CLICKER TRAINING

A 'conditioned reinforcer' is a stimulus which holds no particular significance for a dog until it is closely associated or paired with something highly significant, such as food. A dog does not need to learn the significance of food, which is therefore an 'unconditioned reinforcer'. If the significance of a stimulus has to be learned, it is termed 'conditioned'. Once this linking of events is established, the conditioned reinforcer has the same rewarding and emotional effect as food itself and can be used to pinpoint desirable behaviours. In turn, specific words can be added to the learning curve, which later function as commands.

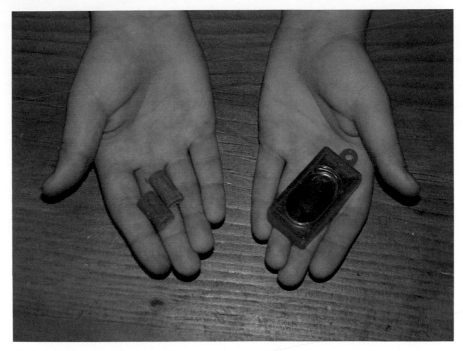

Clicker and food.

The tool which has become widely and effectively used in this way is the 'clicker', a device making a sound not heard in any other context. Once it is closely linked by multiple repetitions with the imminent arrival of food (the dog has become 'clicker aware'), the sound itself reinforces behaviour. Importantly, it becomes a sound the dog positively wants to hear and will be attended to preferentially. It can therefore be used in the face of other auditory distractions and, seemingly paradoxically, for many sound-sensitive dogs.

The principles of clicker training are, however, frequently misunderstood and the device misused. The clicker used properly involves both *associative* (or classical) and *operant* conditioning. Firstly, the classical Pavlovian association between sound and food must be firmly established. Secondly, the dog must do something in order to receive a 'click and treat' (hence operant conditioning). The trainer must therefore wait until the dog performs a predetermined specific behaviour before delivering reward. The choice of behaviour is the dog's. When to click is in the hands of the trainer.

Herein lie the commonly made mistakes. A dog coming running to his owner when he hears the click is simply associating the sound with delivery of food and it has therefore become a recall cue replacing the verbal 'Come here!' He assumes that he must be at his owner's feet in order for the food to be obtained and that he must therefore approach his owner very quickly. He has not learned which specific behaviour made the click happen. Take the 'sit' at a distance from the owner as an example. If the dog sits when asked, the 'sit' is clicked. The dog must then stay sitting while the owner approaches to deliver food. The sequence should be 'desirable behaviour', then 'click', then 'deliver reward'.

It is interesting to think that, had Pavlov made the 'sit' a behavioural requirement before ringing the bell and presenting food to his dogs, his experiment would be held up as an example of both *associative* and *operant* conditioning.

I often find myself thinking of behaviours as pin numbers. In 'clicker training' parlance, a dog will 'offer' behaviours in order to find out which of them will gain the reward of a 'click and treat'. An imaginative risk-taking dog, often considered troublesome, may be the best candidate for clicker training, offering many behaviours quickly in succession (a stand, sit, paw up, circle, pick up a sock, etc.) until we select the one we want.

By the same token, we may have multiple credit or debit cards in our wallet and sometimes have to find the correct number by trial and error in order to satisfy the cash machine and gain the 'reward' of cash. We need to be as crystal clear as cash point technology if we are not to confuse canine companions.

'CASH IN HAND' VERSUS 'PAYSLIP'

To continue the monetary theme and comparing obedience to paid for human work, I often think that dogs can be split into two categories: those of 'cash in hand' and of 'payslip' dogs. In the former, obedience is the equivalent of cash in hand labour. Cash is offered and may have to be seen before a job is agreed to be carried out. In the latter, work is done in the trust that remuneration will arrive in the bank as promised by the payslip.

A frequent complaint among dog owners is that their dog will obey a command only if food is shown to the dog first. What is happening of course is that the dog has been given no reliable and consistent reason to obey unless a tangible incentive – food – is seen at the start. It is this phenomenon which leads to accusations of 'bribery and corruption' in dog training.

In puppy training or for difficult adult tasks, food may well be needed as a lure. But the cash in hand expectation can and should be gradually replaced by the canine payslip. Such cash in hand dogs (of which there are many) have simply never been given the opportunity to realise and trust that their reward will arrive even if not seen first. By an owner patiently waiting until the dog performs a desired action before producing food (as in clicker training), a dog can grow to trust that money will be in the bank after the work is done. Only then can they be termed pay-slip dogs.

OBEDIENCE VERSUS WELL-BEHAVEDNESS

It is very easy for 'obedience' to be confused with 'well-behavedness' and *vice versa*. Well-behaved dogs may rarely cause their owners any trouble. They do not jump up at visitors, fight with other dogs or run away from their owners in the park. The behaviours performed are all the dog's idea but they just happen to be convenient to their owner. In truth, well-behavedness simply means 'absence of bad'. Such dogs may be very easy to live with and require very little in the way of obedience training. But if asked to do something they haven't already decided to do, they may in reality not be very obedient at all.

On the other hand, dogs may be highly obedience trained. They may win prizes in obedience competitions and, with their handler, be held up as role models for other owners and their dogs to emulate. But if these dogs are left to their own devices, they may be all at sea without instruction and make all the wrong decisions.

Owners need to be made aware of this distinction and strike a happy medium between the two. To get rid of all canine foibles would rid them of their charm and the reason that one 'guilty' look enables them to wrap us around their metaphorical 'little finger'. Too many misdemeanours ill-advisedly dealt with and the whole relationship may be at risk. The average pet dog owner does not need advanced training for his or her dog. A reliable 'come here', 'sit' and 'lie down' will suffice for most day-to-day purposes. The rest of the time, the dog should be allowed to be a dog. To chase the odd ball, chew the odd bone and do what they do best – watch the world go by and sleep.

SUMMARY

1. What a dog does is always his own choice, not ours.
2. It is based upon what he feels he has to do (an experience-based cost-benefit analysis of outcomes of behaviour).
3. An obedient dog is working upon exactly the same principles as a disobedient one.
4. An obedience command is a means of giving a dog the information it needs upon which to base its decision.
5. Obedience must be distinguished from well-behavedness.
6. A dog acting out of willing choice will not need to become aggressive.

CONCLUSION

Dogs are continually trying to fit in with human society as they have done for millennia. To achieve this, they have to appear to do as we want them to. An obedient animal is therefore on every dog owner's wish list. But for a mutually satisfying relationship to exist, we must also appear to fulfil a dog's wishes. Problems arise when the expectations of the relationship on either side do not meet its provisions. Obedience, properly defined, understood and humanely instilled, can rectify certain relational shortcomings but only in part. We should also give dogs the time and space just to be themselves without requiring anything of them. Our needs must not take total precedence over theirs, nor should we pander to every apparent canine whim. Our aim must be to create an honest, healthy and mutually happy relationship.

> The single biggest problem with communication is the illusion that it has taken place.
>
> George Bernard Shaw

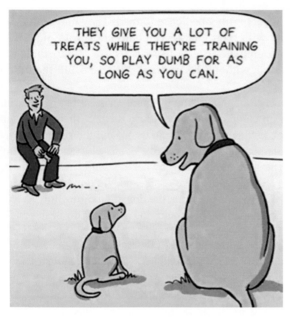

BREVITY © 2011 Dist. By ANDREWS MCMEEL SYNDICATION. Reprinted with permission. All rights reserved.

Part II

Dogs and owners

5 The Ladder of Aggression

THE HISTORY OF THE LADDER OF AGGRESSION

Around 2000, Professor Daniel Mills of Lincoln University Life Sciences Department asked if I would write a chapter on social behaviour and communication in dogs for a new publication – the first edition of a behavioural medicine manual for veterinary surgeons to be published by the British Small Animal Veterinary Association (BSAVA). I accepted this invitation with some trepidation, particularly as I was not his first choice (Dr. Ian Dunbar having declined), realising as I did that it would entail much unaccustomed reading and referencing. The chapter was eventually entitled 'Development of behaviour, social behaviour and communication in the dog' and the manual, covering both dogs and cats, was published in 2002.

By the time of writing the chapter, I had already formulated some of my own ideas about how and why dogs expressed themselves, particularly with regard to peace-keeping gestures, and had been considerably influenced by Turid Rugaas and what she termed 'calming signals' (1997). I had long questioned the relevance of the concepts of 'dominance' and 'submission' as they were then routinely applied to canine body language and had wondered whether the average dog would agree with this historical wisdom. At worst, these terms were being applied as if dominance and submission were fixed features of an individual, akin to being large or black, rather than 'this dog is behaving in a dominant or submissive manner'. And yet it was self-evident that there was a fluidity between communicative gestures and that a dog who may have appeared to be the epitome of submission one minute could become mountainously dominant the next. Yet I could find nothing in the literature at that time to officially support what I wanted to say.

The closest I could get was to the concept of 'resource holding potential' as a means of resolving conflicts (Parker 1974) which basically accepted that if a resource was considered extremely valuable by one individual, and a second did not care enough to be potentially injured over it, the latter would appear to concede defeat. In most cases, possession appeared to be '9/10ths of the law': 'it's mine and you're not having it'. Rather than understanding that resource value was the determining factor in the interaction, an observer might have his entrenched opinion reinforced, that one individual was showing dominance over the other submissive animal. In turn, dogs that growled at their owners over a bone or food bowl were, and still are, labelled as dominant to be dealt with accordingly.

But was this really the whole story?

In researching the chapter, I came across a diagram illustrating 'expressive social responses in the dog' attributed to Fox and Bekoff 1975 and cited in K. Houpt's

Domestic Animal Behaviour for Veterinarians in 1982. The schema indicated a one-way transition between gestures and that both play-soliciting and a more aggressive stance could move towards a fearful and so-called submissive posture. Submission was moreover subdivided into *active*, when some movement was being performed by a dog to indicate its submissive state, and *passive*, when a dog was frozen into inactivity.

I could not accept these interpretations knowing as I did from practical experience how a very still 'frozen' dog might prove to be far more likely to bite if mismanaged than a dog raising a paw and licking its nose. Likewise a dog lying down with a rear leg raised could not be trusted to tolerate a tummy tickle from all comers. I therefore had the illustrations redrawn and took the liberty of having them relabelled omitting any mention of dominance or submission, active or passive. Instead, as can be seen, I subdivided the postures into signals which indicated a dog was content with distance *decreasing* between them and another individual and those which clearly showed that an *increase* in distance was being requested. When put in the context of a human-dog interaction, it is these requests for more space, particularly if subtle, that are so often ignored or misinterpreted with injurious consequences.

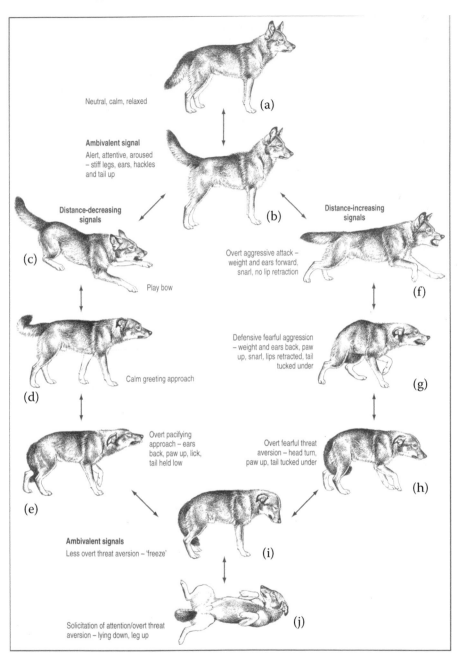

Neutral, calm, relaxed (a)

Ambivalent signal
Alert, attentive, aroused
– stiff legs, ears, hackles
and tail up (b)

Distance-decreasing signals (c)

Distance-increasing signals

Overt aggressive attack –
weight and ears forward,
snarl, no lip retraction (f)

Play bow

Defensive fearful aggression
– weight and ears back, paw
up, snarl, lips retracted, tail
tucked under (g)

Calm greeting approach (d)

Overt pacifying
approach – ears
back, paw up, lick,
tail held low (e)

Overt fearful threat
aversion – head turn,
paw up, tail tucked under (h)

Ambivalent signals
Less overt threat aversion – 'freeze' (i)

Solicitation of attention/overt threat
aversion – lying down, leg up (j)

Expressive social responses in the dog. (Redrawn after Fox and Bekoff, 1975. Reproduced with permission from the BSAVA Manual of Canine and Feline Behavioural Medicine, 1st Edition © BSAVA.)

Meanwhile, all these thoughts seemed to coalesce and support a concept in diagrammatic form which I had begun to construct and had termed the 'Ladder of

Aggression'. It showed in a linear fashion how a dog might move up the metaphorical ladder if subtle 'polite' signals were not responded to appropriately (you could call the response 'rudeness') and on up towards threatened or overt aggression. Even worse was for gestures to be met, not simply by rudeness or lack of social nicety, but by threat, so that the exact opposite of what was intended, that of maintaining harmony, was the result. I also realised that dogs were continually moving up and down the ladder according to context, all the while trying to avoid biting. Very much thinking along the lines of 'publish and be damned', the diagram was submitted for inclusion in the BSAVA manual chapter and, somewhat to my surprise, was accepted by the editors.

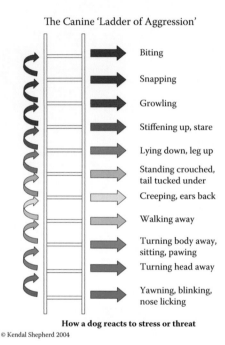

The Canine 'Ladder of Aggression'

Biting

Snapping

Growling

Stiffening up, stare

Lying down, leg up

Standing crouched, tail tucked under

Creeping, ears back

Walking away

Turning body away, sitting, pawing

Turning head away

Yawning, blinking, nose licking

How a dog reacts to stress or threat

© Kendal Shepherd 2004

Reproduced with permission from the *BSAVA Manual of Canine and Feline Behavioural Medicine*, 1st Edition © BSAVA.

The rest, as they say, is history. As well as being published in 2002, the Ladder of Aggression appeared in the second edition of the manual in 2009 and was lavishly illustrated by the late Magy Howard. It is available in poster form from BSAVA Publications.

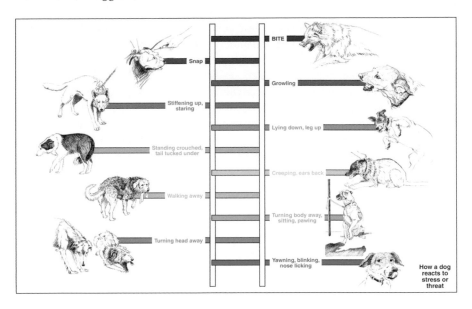

The text accompanying the diagram in the 2009 BSAVA manual reads:

The Ladder of Aggression is a depiction of the gestures that any dog will give in response to an escalation of perceived stress and threat, from very mild social interaction and pressure, to which blinking and nose licking are appropriate responses, to severe, when overt aggression may well selected. The purpose of such behaviour is to deflect threat and restore harmony and the presence of appeasing and threat-averting behaviour in the domestic dog's repertoire is essential to avoid the need for potentially damaging aggression. The dog is a social animal for whom successful appeasement behaviour is highly adaptive and it is used continually and routinely in every-day life. It is most important to realise that these gestures are simply a context and response-dependant sequence which will culminate in threatened or overt aggression, only if all else fails.

Contrary to persistent misinformation, the gestures identified are nothing to do with a purported dominant or submissive state relative to companions. In all dogs, inappropriate social responses to appeasement behaviour will result in its devaluing and the necessity, from a dog's perspective, to move up the ladder. Aggression is therefore created in any situation where appeasement behaviour is chronically misunderstood and not effective in obtaining the socially expected outcome. Dogs may progress to overt aggression within seconds during a single episode if the perceived threat occurs quickly and at close quarters, or learn to dispense with lower rungs on the ladder over time, if repeated efforts to appease are misunderstood and responded to inappropriately. As a consequence, a so-called 'unpredictable' aggressive response, without any obvious preamble, may occur in any context which predicts inescapable threat to the dog, when in reality it was entirely predictable.

(Shepherd, 2009, pp. 3–6)

Canine appeasement behaviour would seem to be the linchpin upon which the dog-human relationship revolves in that dogs have been, and still are being, strongly selected for the appearance that appeasement behaviour embodies. We love dogs which look like they love us (see Chapter 1). There is therefore a profound significance for our relationship with them, as well as for the welfare of dogs themselves, if appeasement behaviour which has been so crucial to the evolution of the dog is chronically misunderstood and devalued. From the dog's perspective, it is as if the evolutionary goalposts have been seismically shifted. If appeasement behaviour no longer appears to serve its purpose, it is as radical a change as the giraffe having suddenly to eat off the floor and its long neck and legs becoming redundant.

We now recognise that biting is not an aberration or deviation from the norm but part of any dog's normal behavioural repertoire. The canine world is not divided into 'nice' dogs who would never bite no matter what and 'vicious' dogs who do so at the drop of a hat. The tolerance of human behaviour that dogs show, the give and take that exists in any relationship, does, however, vary so much that we may be easily misled into imagining that dogs exist in these two categories. Selection for certain behavioural traits will affect how readily an individual moves towards aggression. Breeds selected for their reactivity and ability to respond in an instant to obedience cues will prove to be very useful in certain contexts but may be condemned as dangerous in others when the same level of reactivity is applied to human misunderstanding of their body language.

SIGNIFICANCE AND USE OF THE LADDER OF AGGRESSION IN PRACTISE

The Ladder of Aggression, in summary, depicts an escalation of appeasing and threat-averting gestures towards overt aggression, which have the single aim of maintaining or restoring harmony. If appeasement behaviour does not work, either during one incident or over a period of time, aggression will inevitably result. When explaining the ladder to clients, it is important to point out that the more subtle signs on the bottom rungs are the equivalent of polite human social gestures, such as the handshake or smile. Just as we would not want to be hugged or kissed or even touched by everyone we happen to smile at, these subtle gestures must be taken in the context in which they are given and not interpreted as *carte blanche* permission for anyone to do as they like.

THE FOUR FS

The ways in which a dog may respond to threat have also been termed 'the four Fs'. These are alliteratively divided into the **flight**, **fight**, **freeze** and **faff-about**. 'Fight' and 'flight' are fairly unambiguous—as long as it is fully understood that prevention of 'flight' will inevitably result in 'fight'. We are all familiar with the phrase 'frozen with fear' and are aware that the state of being frozen may convert to either fight or flight in both humans and dogs, depending on perceived need and behavioural options available.

The 'faff-about' mode of dealing with stress and threat is, however, readily misinterpreted. The over-excited dog who seems for all the world so pleased to see us and the puppy wriggling, licking and wagging its tail madly on the consulting room table may instead be deploying this tactic to express unease and insecurity in these contexts. They may be equally prepared to snap and bite should they be misunderstood. The temptation to respond with forceful restraint to keep the dog still is no doubt very great. Please resist it! Equally importantly, do not reciprocate in kind to the apparent greeting and 'fuss' the dog. Allowing time for the dog to calm down by ignoring such excesses, then proceeding to use well-rehearsed obedience commands before commencing any 'hands on' procedure is a far better approach.

RESOURCE GUARDING

A 'resource guarder' is a term frequently used to describe a dog who threatens aggression when an object is in his possession and someone (either a dog or human) comes too close and appears to want it too. Such prized objects commonly include food, its bowl, toys, the sofa, a dog's bed and, of course, the fabled bone. Consequently, the label 'possessive aggression' is used to describe the behaviour. Stolen objects, such as shoes, may be fun to chew, but are also inadvertently made more valuable in a dog's eyes by the attention we give to thieving behaviour and because we inevitably try to retrieve our footwear.

It must be stressed here that dogs do not use aggression to *gain* a resource but to guard and *maintain* possession only, although they may well use other more subtle ways to get what they want. This may seem less than obvious to begin with, but we could never have developed the relationship we have with dogs if they were prepared to attack us for anything they happened to want. Instead, the food treat in our pocket is in our undisputed possession and can therefore be used as a bargaining tool. However, there can be a fine perceptual line as to when and where something leaves our possession and becomes 'owned' by a dog. The dog's dinner is a prime example. It is obvious to all that once the bowl is on the floor and the dog's nose is in it, the dinner is his. Any perceived attempt to remove it may be met with vigorous objection. But does the bowl have to be actually on the ground before guarding is thought justified? Does it even have to have any food in it? It is obvious that hands reaching down towards the bowl predict loss of a resource and may trigger aggression. It is less immediately obvious that feet being too close, or even if someone is merely in the kitchen at the same time, can come to predict possible loss as well and have the same result. In this way, a dog's 'sphere of influence' may increase in both time and space and guarding behaviour become justified.

Less common is for aggression shown at other times and in other places to be considered as simply an expression of 'resource guarding'. Instead, alternative labels are created which imply context: for example, territorial aggression describes a dog who may bark and growl at the postman or other passers-by and maternal aggression, a bitch who defends her puppies. The dog who defends the family from visitors (intruders in the dog's eyes), or indeed one family member from another, may be fondly thought of as being 'protective', with all this word's ambivalent implications. A dog running away with and defending a stolen shoe is simply 'disobedient' or 'naughty'.

A dog becoming aggressive (over time or in an instant) on veterinary handling would never typically be described as a resource guarder, but the most vital resource they (and people for that matter) possess are their own body parts. In order to make full use of the interpretive value of the Ladder of Aggression, it is far simpler to get rid of labels, at least in one's own mind, and consider that these gestures will be expressed when *anything* a dog values is thought to be under threat.

Whether aggression is selected immediately or other more subtle 'polite' communicative gestures are tried first will depend on the degree and proximity of threat posed, as well as the dog's past experience of what works in reducing or repelling threat. All too often, aggression is thought to come out of the blue because subtle signs are misinterpreted or not noticed at all. A dog walking away with a toy or stolen item rather than obeying a 'come here' command is not showing a reckless disregard for authority but responding in the way evolution has dictated.

Another vital factor to be taken into account is whether a resource can be moved by the dog or not. A bone can; the sofa cannot. A ball or stolen shoe can be run away with; a favoured place to lie, such as a doorway, cannot. A dog's body is usually movable but restraint on lead will force a change of tactic from walking away (lower down on the ladder) to more overt defence (higher up). We will all recognise the dog pulling towards the exit to avoid our attentions yet being held tightly on lead and pulled back.

Overt aggression is rarely a dog's first option – unless experience has inadvertently taught the dog that it is the *only* option. The risk of a dog feeling the need for aggressive defence may be ameliorated by giving *more choice* as to what to do rather than less. This may well seem counterintuitive. How many alternatives are available? Is the sofa the only really comfortable place to lie in the house? Has the dog his own toys in the house? If so, they must be made to seem valuable by being treated by the owners as if they were indeed a stolen shoe, if chewing toys rather than shoes is to be preferred. Is the consulting room door and pulling towards it the only apparent means of getting to safety?

In general, the dog is more likely to bite if threats increase and resources and behavioural options decrease. A simple equation may therefore be used both to analyse previous aggressive episodes and to help to predict and pre-empt future events:

Threats↑ + resources↓ + behavioural options ↓ = aggressive response↑

Alternatively,

Threats↓ + resources↑ + behavioural options ↑ = aggressive response↓

In essence, the more behavioural options and the greater the number of resources a dog has, together with the fewer perceived threats the dog experiences, the less likely the need for aggression becomes.

Reducing perceived threat, devaluing resources (by giving more of them) and increasing behavioural options reduces the likelihood of a bite. It follows that if a dog bites with no identifiable or predictable threat, no resources to guard other than its own body and with all behavioural options readily available, such a dog is truly dangerous.

THE CONTRIBUTION OF PAIN

We ignore pain at our peril. Dogs that predict pain and discomfort on trying to move away from a threat will prevent retreat just as surely as restraint. Any dog that is displaying aggression in any context, but particularly if apparent resource guarding (including the dog's own body) has become an issue, should be thoroughly examined for any pain. This is particularly vital where breed-related skeletal conditions are prevalent. We must be aware that dogs may be in pain for some considerable time before limping is evident as a physical symptom. **Aggression is a vitally important early behavioural symptom of pain and should not be ignored.**

THE CASE OF CHILLI

As we know from our own experience, pain can make anyone short-tempered and tetchy, but how pain and environment could combine to specifically convert 'flight' to 'fight' was brought home to me shortly after the publication of the Ladder of Aggression. A five-year-old female Border Collie called Chilli suffering with bilateral hip dysplasia was being considered for surgery. Matters had come to a head with refusal of a total hip joint replacement by an orthopaedic specialist, on the grounds of her 'unacceptable' (in other words extremely aggressive) behaviour during examination. Chilli was therefore in the ultimate Catch-22 situation, having been refused a procedure to relieve her of pain because of her aggression, but unlikely to improve very much behaviourally until suffering considerably less pain.

Hip dysplasia had been diagnosed during her first year of life and the very severe nature of this condition recently confirmed. All aggressive episodes had been triggered by the possibility that she might have to stand up and move. When younger, her response to unwelcome attention consisted simply of grumbling and moving away. Her physical problems had also become the excuse for her behaviour in the owners' minds. The family had tolerated and condoned her frequent 'air snaps' towards them on being touched, and towards visitors who attempt to interact with her, for most of her life. Chilli's air snaps had therefore become firmly engrained as a successful and pain-relieving strategy.

Chilli's behaviour had, however, deteriorated since the owners' house move 18 months previously. She had progressed from snapping to actual biting. It was most revealing to be told that there was a significant difference between the two houses. In comparison with fully fitted carpets previously, there was only laminate flooring downstairs in the new house, which had made getting to and keeping her feet much harder and more painful for Chilli than it used to be.

I supplied a Ladder of Aggression diagram to remind the owners of all the gestures dogs use to demonstrate unease and to avert threat. Over the years, Chilli had dispensed with the lower rungs as unreliable and, on veterinary examination, jumped immediately to the top of the ladder. Their task was to revalue the lower and non-aggressive rungs on the ladder by making sure Chilli's gestures were understood and responded to correctly. Of particular importance was to realise that the typical 'guilty' look was actually appeasement behaviour designed to stop us being cross and threatening. Anytime this behaviour was ignored (often seemingly of necessity at the vets) or misinterpreted, aggression became more likely.

SUMMARY

I have found the Ladder of Aggression concept and diagram a most useful tool to illustrate the gestures owners can so clearly recognise in their own dogs. I am extremely gratified that, since its translation into various languages, it has proved essential to so many trainers and behaviourists worldwide. Understanding the true significance of the gestures and their context-specific nature is crucial to avoid dogs being pushed into displaying overt aggression.

6 How to 'speak client'

This chapter covers
How to interpret what a client is saying about the pet's behaviour
The choice and use of words
'Treat' versus reward
What does 'good' mean in behavioural terms

When any verbal history is taken regarding the problem behaviour of a dog, words will be used by owners to give their view on what a dog does, why they do it and, by implication, what their ideal expectations of their dog are. These words are usually laden with anthropomorphic overtones. They may be used very much as a parent will speak to, or about, a child and are therefore a reflection of how dogs have been viewed and incorporated into the human family. The phrases may even be spoken to lighten the mood by way of a rather embarrassed apology for a dog's misbehaviour.

Although anthropomorphism has enhanced the dog-human relationship in many respects, the language used often reflects fundamental misunderstandings in the relationship which can be very damaging in practical terms. Unravelling the language used, and why, is enormously helpful in understanding an owner's perception and attitude as well as giving informed guidance as how to address his or her concerns during any consultation. Descriptions such as being 'stubborn', 'having a mind of his own', being 'strong-willed' and 'disobedient' as well as 'deciding he knows better that me' are all too common. Ubiquitous beliefs that the dog is 'bossy' or 'too dominant' are fed by apparently authoritative, but mistaken, media figures. Equally, in a legal context, such phrases may be used to describe and condemn a dog in court. Magistrates may be equally susceptible to anthropomorphism when the prosecution is alleging 'dangerousness'.

The following are all commonly heard phrases. They are not intended to spark a detailed lecture given to the client regarding the tacit fallacies entailed. But briefly untangling in one's own mind what they are trying to say, if not in theirs, may be very beneficial. If a dog is asked to sit with food and an upward moving hand by demonstration rather than by detailed explanation in response to a dog being told to 'Behave yourself!', the message may gradually filter through.

'BEHAVE!'

I love this! 'Behave' is used as a command word as if a dog is supposed to know what the word means and, more importantly, what to do. As ever, it is uttered when a dog is misbehaving and therefore is very rarely in a jolly tone of voice. It does not inform anyone, least of all the dog, as to what they *should* do but only what they should *not* be doing. The means whereby information (such as it is) has been imparted will be by an owner's demeanour, incorporating both vocal expression and body gestures. If the dog is on lead, a leash jerk or collar grab may accompany the vocal admonishment. If the dog is supposed to be sitting or standing, the hindquarters may be pushed downwards or pulled upwards as required. The only clue a dog may have as to an acceptable behaviour is when the nagging and disapproval and physical prompts stop. There is also a distinct danger that the word, being randomly linked to whatever a dog is doing and feeling at the time, will have the opposite effect to what is intended. If used as a warning of worse to come if a dog does not 'behave', the very sound of the word may trigger negative emotions.

'HE'S SO STUBBORN'

Stubbornness is defined in the Oxford English dictionary as 'having or showing dogged determination not to change one's attitude or position on something, especially in spite of good reasons to do so'. It may be considered the antithesis of **biddable** which describes someone 'meekly ready to accept and follow instructions' or 'willing to obey and to do what they are told to'. 'Biddable' is commonly used to describe the dog who is easy to train, often not needing food to be shown what to do and rarely putting a foot wrong. They are the envy of owners of 'stubborn' dogs, who may be led to believe by such shining examples that they and their dog are abject failures on the training front.

But what does being 'biddable', and by contrast, 'stubborn', actually mean? Are they reflections of how much effort has been put into training, or of the fundamental nature of the dog in question itself? I would suggest that biddable describes a dog who is very aware of human displeasure and consequently easily guided by the mildest of rebukes. A mere frown accompanied by 'Oi!' is sufficient to make a dog stop and think again. They may be particularly aware of human upset, which, if it is directly linked to a dog's behaviour, is sufficiently unpleasant (therefore punishing) to them that they will avoid doing the same in the future. Guide dogs are specifically selected for a biddable nature and even causing a person to stumble during training may be enough to punish a wrong move.

On the opposite side of the coin, there is the stubborn dog who appears to resist all efforts to change the decision he has made. He seems immune to persuasion, whether by promise of reward or threat of punishment.

Could these differences be caused not only by degree of sensitivity to human emotion but also by how prepared a dog is to take risks? As with people, the degree of risk involved in any activity is overcome by the desire to engage in it. The feeling of exhilaration, elation and frank relief that is experienced once the fear of engaging in an extreme sport is conquered successfully is highly rewarding and can become addictive. In a similar fashion, some dogs appear almost deliberately to put themselves into positions certain to incur human wrath and punishment. Why? Because the punishment itself and its administration provides an extremely potent negative reward when it ceases. They therefore become addicted to the emotion of relief once the unpleasantness ends.

'HE HAS A MIND OF HIS OWN!'

Suppressing one's instinctive but possibly belittling response, 'Whose mind is he supposed to have then?', may be extremely difficult. What is often spoken in jest is, of course, quite obviously true. It is necessary to understand why this phrase is so commonly heard and what it is about a dog that warrants such a description. A dog which has a mind of his own seems otherwise at risk of being condemned as having a faulty brain and outlook on life. Yet all that is actually happening is simply that the dog's choice of behaviour is often at odds with that of his owner's.

Frustrated as owners may be with their dogs' 'wilfulness', it is necessary to clarify the phrase and to explain that, like an apparently 'stubborn' dog, some personalities and temperaments, or 'minds', may prove more challenging to change than others. Owners may feel they have to work hard to get the dog's own choice of behaviour to coincide with their own. But it is far easier to avoid conflict altogether. Simply spending more time deliberately noticing and approving of their 'stubborn' dog when he is already doing what they would like, will do the trick. Dogs are often ignored when resting, lying down calmly, when the lead happens to be slack on a walk or when the dog is looking at them rather than at other distractions. Noticing and approving of such voluntarily performed 'good' behaviours will do much to improve the relationship between dog and owner. Owners will also come to realise that dogs do indeed have minds of their own!

'HE'S SO GLAD TO BE HERE!'

Assuming a dog is 'happy' to enter the surgery is a risky assumption at best. It is often not recognised that the excited panting dog with wagging tail pulling his owner into the waiting or consulting room is actually showing signs of stress and insecurity. As such, they may be as intolerant of handling and restraint as the more obviously fearful animal. Excitement may be compounded by the owner fussing the dog and even inviting others to do the same. Do not be afraid to appear to be rude and ignore the dog. Explain to the client that this is not how truly happy dogs behave and that paying attention at such times, however much the dog may appear to want it, will only perpetuate the behaviour.

Ask in how many other contexts such excitement is seen. Often wild excesses of greeting behaviour (jumping up, pawing and licking) are interpreted as demonstrating a dog's delight in welcoming visitors. They should not reciprocate if the dog is to be allowed to become confident and calm.

'HE USED TO BE FINE!'

I was once discussing this particular phrase (often uttered by clients with a degree of puzzlement) with Dr. Roger Mugford. In his inimitable fashion, he commented, 'He also used to be four months old!' Although this was stating the obvious, the saying highlights that whereas age changes, the expectation is often that behaviour ought to stay the same. It is not realised that good behaviour needs nurturing if it is not to wither and die.

It also may help to point out how mature a 4-month-old puppy is, and that in human terms they are already the developmental equivalent of a 5-year-old child.

They are not the babies fondly imagined, and much formative learning should have occurred before a puppy is presented for first vaccination.

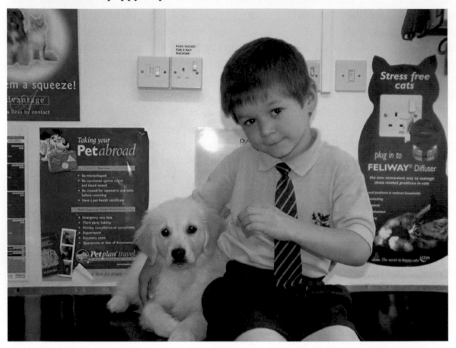

A 5-year-old child already knows how to say please and thank you and where they should go to the loo. Yet puppies often have vital social lessons still to learn at the equivalent developmental age. These lessons should have begun much earlier. Pleasant handling by strangers of both sexes, adults as well as children, should ideally begin before the puppy leaves the litter and continue many times afterwards. In this way, what may be considered as a 'bank of trust' is built up whereby the puppy may in effect forgive a later unpleasantness.

The concept of **latent inhibition** is that it is often easier to learn something new than to unlearn something familiar. Any previous experiences may be thought of as being stored in a bank and which are not easily forgotten. Any new experience is, however, quickly learned and remembered. It is essential therefore that all experiences are made as pleasant as possible and repeated many times. A quickly learned new experience which may be unpleasant will be offset against the bank of pleasant memories. It will thus have far less significance if many stored pleasant memories exist.

If, however, the bank of pleasant memories is lacking or not great enough, there is nothing to set a new unpleasant experience against. A single unpleasantness will be sufficient to create a long-lasting memory in the same context. In this way, the dog that used to be 'fine' becomes increasingly distrustful over time.

'HE JUST DOESN'T LISTEN!'

*My daughter was a rather bright three-year old when, one afternoon, I was at-
tempting to call her in from the garden for tea. Engrossed as she was in playing, she
appeared to be ignoring me entirely. After a short while, to my surprise and not a
little consternation, she announced emphatically that she couldn't possibly come in
because she was deaf.*

*This caused me some considerable pause for thought. After all, I didn't think at
this age she even knew the meaning of the word. As it turned out, she didn't.*

*I slowly came to the realisation that I was in the habit of saying, if being ignored,
'Are you deaf?!', usually after several repetitions of a request in an increasingly
irritated tone of voice.*

*She therefore, being indeed ignorant of the word's true meaning, assumed that
'deaf' must be what she was under such circumstances. Surely she must be. I had
called her it often enough. I had of course taught her an obvious, but in reality
entirely erroneous, lesson.*

How often do we instil the same faulty lesson in our dogs? Words heard si-
multaneously with a performed behaviour can only become mentally attached by
the dog (or young child) to that particular behaviour. Dogs have no capacity to
interpret words to mean something that we'd prefer them to be doing at some time
in the future. Repeating 'Come here!' to a dog rapidly disappearing in the opposite
direction in an increasingly exasperated tone of voice makes it unlikely that a dog
will think that running to, instead of away from an angry owner is the sensible
choice. This also runs the real risk of causing 'behavioural deafness'.

'HE DOESN'T REALLY MEAN IT!'

This is most commonly uttered either in the consulting room after a dog has
growled or snapped or during a behaviour consultation to excuse a dog that has a
history of doing so. The reason this belief exists is because of the way a dog will
typically behave immediately after growling or snapping. This is to show appeasing
behaviour (aka the 'guilty' look), in turn accepted by the owner as an acknowledgement of wrongdoing and interpreted as an apology. What then mystifies owners
is why, if a dog is indeed so sorry, he continues to repeat the same mistake over and
over again in the same context. Surely he should learn not to do it again?

Of course, any dog which growls or snaps does mean it, and very sincerely at that.
The context in which growling or snapping occurs must be examined thoroughly in order
to discover what provoked the behaviour and what response it received. If the growl or
snap is successful in repelling threat, a dog will express relief with appeasing behaviour to
try to ensure the apparent conflict does not resume. If not, then a dog may progress to
biting in earnest.

Clients must be disabused of any notion that a dog does not mean what he does
or indeed does anything without reason. Dogs do not pretend. If the trigger for
growling or snapping is the owner's angry response to a misdemeanour of some
kind, the threat the owners themselves pose must cease immediately. If not, a dog

will be pushed towards biting. This is irrespective of how instinctive and justified their actions may seem. Impress on them that they are not giving in to the dog, simply indicating their understanding of him and keeping themselves safe (see Chapter 5 'The Ladder of Aggression').

'HE DOESN'T NEED FOOD!'

I heard this from an 'old school' Jack Russell owner as he lifted his dog onto the table by collar one end and stump of tail at the other. I gave the dog a piece of food anyway, thereby risking further owner disapproval. But why this attitude? It all stems from the belief that food is simply a temptation or treat and somehow spoils a dog. Using the word 'payment' rather than 'treat', even without further explanation, helps to chip away at such notions. Simply standing on a vet's table is a task hard enough for a dog to warrant recompense. 'He doesn't need food' is also a reflection of how convinced this owner was that his dog would not dare to misbehave and, in turn, might give an idea of how 'obedience' had been instilled in the past. I strongly suspected that threatened or real punishment was the sole means whereby this little dog had 'learned his lessons'.

The following case incorporates many of these confusions and misinterpretations and illustrates how they can be resolved. It also acts as a fitting summary and conclusion to this chapter.

Jed was a 2½-year-old male working Cocker Spaniel showing supposed 'dominance aggression' towards his owners over stolen items. It illustrates how crucial it is to tease out accurate interpretation and meaning of phrases and descriptions used by the owners to ensure mutual understanding and to restore the dog's trust in them.

The owners' wish, stated in the pre-consultation questionnaire, was that their dog would 'understand that we are in charge' and that 'asking for compliance with the rules does not mean he is losing face'. They also wanted him to 'love himself' and sincerely wished for him to be 'happy'. Most pertinently, they realised that Jed was behaving for much of the time 'as if he was unsure of what was going on'.

These interpretations of how their dog was feeling and how his emotions were thought to impact on his behaviour were unusually mindful and descriptive. I was intrigued, particularly as the use of an electric shock collar to discourage running off on walks seemed at odds with the wish that he should be happy. It was also illuminating to find that a second Cocker bitch in the family was no longer deemed suitable for work as she 'wouldn't do what she was told'. The fact that she 'had a mind of her own' was considered a fault.

How these phrases were reinterpreted and used to direct the course of the subsequent consultation was vital. The owners, as well as Jed, were utterly confused. They were already familiar with the Ladder of Aggression but at the same time felt that Jed should realise that they had laid down rules which he should follow.

Much of the misunderstanding had its basis in the belief in dominance as a position that dogs strived to gain and that they used aggression to gain it. The client's wish list seemed to encompass this mistaken concept regarding a dog's own perception of status as well as his position in the eyes of others. If he obeyed someone else's rules, he would somehow lose self-esteem. But it was also necessary to clarify the true meaning of obedience. It wasn't simply a matter of telling a dog what to do and expecting him to understand.

Jed had been thought 'biddable' from a young age and had been taught much of what he needed to know by way of a 'threat/no threat' contrast. When Jed had learnt the meaning of the various whistles required by a gun dog, he had tended to be guided by the human approval or disapproval that seemed to result. Although this contrast might work in the majority of situations, it would not suffice when he was in conflict. At times when what his owners wanted him to do was in opposition to what he felt the need to do, he required far clearer and tangible reasons to make his decision. If not, conflict-related aggression was very likely to emerge.

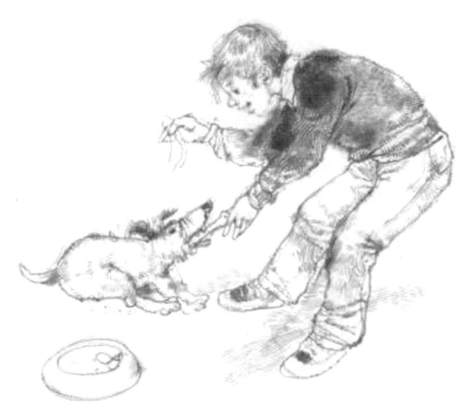

Illustration by Victor Ambrus.

When Jed was caught in the act of stealing, his owners had tended to grab him by his collar, with the intention of forcing him to let go. This is when all the so-called dominantly aggressive bites had occurred. The forceful holding of the collar was threatening in itself and the use of the shock collar had added the prediction of pain to the equation. He had thus become extremely collar shy. He would have been therefore very likely to bite even without the addition of human reprimand.

I was able to convince the owners that all the issues boiled down to three overriding factors. Concentrating on these three would allow their wishes for Jed to be fulfilled.

1. They should rid themselves of any notion that Jed cared two hoots about his social standing.
2. They needed to clear any confusion in their minds regarding what obedience truly meant and how it could be instilled without threat.
3. Jed desperately needed to be clear about exactly how to keep his owners calm. They therefore needed to be clear and consistent.

He could thus attain the state of 'happiness' and self-satisfaction that they so dearly wished for him.

The electric shock collar was voluntarily and swiftly consigned to the bin.

7 Avoiding conflict

PART I AVOIDING CONFLICT BETWEEN DOG AND HUMANS

All that has gone before in this book should, if marked, learned and inwardly digested, result in a better understanding of dogs. It has dealt with their true nature and how they express themselves, what obedience really means and how to ensure they have as good a veterinary experience as possible. If this book has a single aim, it is to reduce the conflict that often seems to exist between our two species, despite the historical ties that bind us inexorably together. Such conflict is most significant if and when misunderstandings result in aggression.

THE 'WHOSE IDEA IS IT?' RULE

Once a dog has begun to threaten aggression, there will have already been countless number of interactions of all kinds between dog and owner. Most of these will have been pleasant and agreeable to both sides. But what about the nagging and grumbles between the parties which occur when a relationship is not at its best? They may have seemed inconsequential at the time and easily resolved. However, such minor disagreements will have a drip-feed effect which may culminate in disaster. Avoiding any routine disagreement is crucial in preventing the emergence of aggression, as well as resolving it once it has become a treatable 'problem'.

The 'Whose idea is it?' rule is a really painless way of avoiding disagreement between dog and owner. If meaningful communication with their pet is established routinely throughout the day, conflict and argument as far as possible can be avoided altogether. This can be achieved by advising clients to follow this rule.

It often seems that dogs are only thought to learn anything when deliberate teaching is being carried out, either in training class or during a training session at home. But dogs, as children, are learning constantly. Many opportunities to teach appropriate lessons, as well as to avoid inappropriate ones, are missed. But any routine interaction between dog and owner has the potential to steer behaviour in the right direction (or conversely the wrong one) whether or not we are conscious of it. Thinking of these interactions as a continuum within the routine day rather than 'we must do some dog training now' ensures that they become an automatic part of life.

Quite simply, the owners should ask themselves, whatever their dog is doing at any time, whose idea was this particular behaviour? In other words, who started it? Is he running about, barking at passers-by, emptying the wastepaper bin or just lying down calmly in his bed? Was the idea theirs or the dog's?

The chances are of course that everything a dog does when at home and not being deliberately 'trained' is his own idea. His idea may or may not be convenient to his owners or indeed socially appropriate. What one can be sure of is that the less-than-desirable, irritating behaviours will always be noticed and reacted to in some way. The far more convenient, calm behaviour will be taken for granted and usually ignored.

Even if noticed, meaningful reward will not be thought necessary. Why on earth reward a dog for what he is already doing of his own volition? Training mantras, such as 'nothing in life is free', tend to leave dog owners with the impression that rewards always have to be earned. Some effort is therefore required on the part of the dog before he can be deemed to be worthy of reward. If he is just lying down, how can that be called work?

But how do we know what a dog has managed to ignore in order to remain calm? A car backfiring, the rattle of the letter box or knock at the door and the telephone ringing may all be obvious to us. But what about sounds of frequencies inaudible to the human ear or so ubiquitous that we have come immune to them? We tend to ignore the central heating turning on or off, the buzz from a laptop, the whirr of the tumble dryer and even the clamour of incessant TV adverts. If a dog is lying down calmly and we want him to remain able to ignore such acoustic intrusions, he needs our meaningful appreciation.

I've never yet been asked for help regarding a dog that was 'too calm'. The dogs causing their owners trouble are often those reactive dogs who seem unable to tell the difference between environmental stimuli that are relevant and meaningful to them (salient) and those of no relevance whatsoever (non-salient). As such almost anything they hear is responded to in an alert and aroused manner. They do not seem to be able to filter out stimuli of little or no importance. Alternatively, non-relevant stimuli have become linked to relevant ones (via associative or classical conditioning) and thus come to generate a similar behavioural response.

The same is true for visual and olfactory stimuli, but when at home, what a dog hears is likely to have the greatest impact. Sound sensitivity is extremely common and may be misdiagnosed as separation anxiety when owners find evidence of canine distress on their return home. The first time a dog experiences a thunderstorm or fireworks, a fearful response may be triggered. Anything in the future that reminds the dog of these events, the weather conditions or time of day or night for example, may result in the same response. If the owners also happened to be absent at the time, then any subsequent departure on their part may trigger the same fear and distress.

If we want calm dogs, then we cannot afford to let calm, non-reactive behaviour pass us by unnoticed and unappreciated. It is when dogs seem to be doing nothing that they need to be given 'something in life for free' if we are to guard against reactivity and promote peacefulness.

The 'Whose idea is it?' rule is simple to follow. Whenever their dog appears relaxed and calm, the owner has two choices:

1. To *reward the calm behaviour* (the dog's idea) by linking praise (i.e. human pleasure) with what he's doing, as in 'Good bed!' or 'Good lie down!' and/or

approach to drop a food treat in front of his nose without saying anything. The aim is that over time the owner will be able to approach and praise the behaviour without the dog moving at all. The calm behaviour should not change but continue as a clear indication of what is required from the dog has been given.

2. To use a calm moment in order to practice *changing the dog's mind* (the owner's idea). Many routine commands and behaviours are simply insufficiently (or never) rehearsed when the dog is calm enough to reliably comply. Asking the dog to 'come here' between different rooms in the house is in effect the rehearsal of recall which, if carried out when the dog is calm to begin with, reduces any risk of conflict and competition with other distractions.

The necessity for approval of the dog behaving calmly of its own volition should also continue outside the house. There are always times on a walk when even the most reactive of dogs is calm. These moments should never be ignored. If the dog is not pulling on lead and not barking, in fact, not doing anything at all other than breathing, walking and maybe looking towards the owner without being asked, a reward should be given automatically. These are also the times when obedience should be rehearsed *before* distractions arise (see also Chapter 9 'The Swimming Pool of Life').

The 'Whose idea is it?' rule summary

To remind you routinely to practise changing your dog's mind in calm, emotionally neutral situations, you must ask yourselves, whatever he is doing and wherever he is, 'Whose idea is it?' The more ideas that become yours, the better control you will have of him.

Alternatively, if your dog is behaving calmly and well without being asked, then make sure you reward him. Never take good behaviour for granted!

Successfully changing the dog's mind throughout the day will imply that you are

- ◦   routinely considering the choices available to your dog
- ◦   making positive requests for 'good' behaviour rather than merely trying to stop the 'bad'
- ◦   using all routine 'life resources', including your attention, to improve your bargaining power
- ◦   rehearsing obedience commands before you need them to work
- ◦   teaching your dog when he is in 'emotional neutral' and finds it easiest to learn
- ◦   not giving in to attention seeking

PART II AVOIDING CONFLICT BETWEEN HUMANS

Chapter 7 covers
Avoiding human-human conflict – how to get arguments resolved
Considering motivation and method to enable behaviour change and satisfy all parties
'Zips theory'

It is so common as to be almost universal that, when eliciting the history of a behaviour problem, one soon uncovers disagreement among family members, mainly between partners, about how the dog should be dealt with and attempts to apportion blame as to whose fault the current state of affairs is. I clearly recall one house visit when I was greeted not with, 'Would you like a coffee before we begin?' but by the female owner vehemently declaring that she would 'get rid of *him* but *never* the dog!'

This calls into question the following:

1. How to get conflicting parties to accept each other's opinion and agree on common means of resolution
2. How to assist in reaching agreement about behaviour modification methods
3. How different motivations and goals can be met by the same means and actions

The answer to probably the most important question posed in my pre-consultation questionnaire, namely, 'Does the dog's behaviour cause arguments at home?' usually forewarns me of any imminent warfare between family members.

Most commonly, these boil down to disagreements about how 'training' of (in other words 'communication with') the dog has been attempted. To cut some very long stories short, it's commonly found that one partner disapproves of the other partner's harsh, disciplinarian approach, whereas the harsh partner will have no patience at all with the first partner's soft, comforting forgiveness of all misdemeanours. Each will be entrenched in their own camp vigorously laying blame on the other for the worsening of their dog's behaviour.

In other cases, thoughts may differ as to why a dog was obtained in the first place. It may be that one partner had to be heavily persuaded against their better judgement to get a dog and has never viewed the new arrival as anything other than a destructive nuisance. The fact problems have arisen justifies their previous misgivings. Subsequent declarations of 'I told you so!' simply rub salt in the wound that the dog's behaviour has caused. One partner may resent the doting attention lavished by the other upon the dog and consider this to be spoiling the dog. By contrast, the doting partner may consider the other to lack feelings for the dog and that they simply do not care.

At this point, it is often necessary to point out that any argument between people may impact on the dog directly, even if it is not about the dog at all. Raised angry voices are extremely upsetting to any dog who may then react in ways which cause further escalation of conflict. The dog may attempt to intervene in the heated exchange by jumping up and even biting. While this is often exceptionally effective in bringing an argument abruptly to an end, accusations such as 'Now look what you'd made him do!' ensue instead. Whatever an argument is about, considering the dog at all times will lead to a quieter and calmer life.

It is often the case that one partner is out at work for much of the day. The fact that they appear absolved from having to deal with a dog's problem behaviour during the day and escape its immediate impact causes resentment. This resentment may be exacerbated by the delight with which the more absent partner is greeted by the dog on their return. It is as if the dog were saying, 'I've had a really horrible time while you were out!'

Occasionally, condemned out of hand by the 'No bad dogs only bad owners' school of thought, an owner would confess, 'I suppose it's all my fault', seemingly expecting my agreement and immediate condemnation. The opinion that all dog are perfect to begin with but get messed up as they get older by ignorant people is unfortunately all too pervasive. I personally have never had any truck with this judgemental attitude, presumably expressed by those whose dogs are perfectly behaved. If I could, I would ask these supposedly exemplary dog owners to 'Let him who is without sin cast the first stone!' We all know owners (including ourselves) who make mistakes while trying to do their best. But we also must accept that there are dogs who would severely tax the patience of a saint.

So how to resolve such arguments without appearing to take sides?

Does it really matter if the reason *why* one party wants resolution differs from the other? It may be that each party has a very valid reason for their opinion. One may well want a cuddly 'happy' dog who doesn't bite above all else, and the other simply need peace and a quiet life with a partner who is not threatening to kick them out of house and home. If they could reach agreement at least about *how* change can be brought about and at the same time acknowledge as valid the motivations of the other, could harmony be restored?

This personal 'light bulb moment' may help.

Zips Theory
Camping as a family has been one of our favourite occupations, despite the vagaries of English weather. It was during one such holiday that I came to an initially puzzling realisation. What had become a routine and mutual niggle between my partner and me at home had virtually disappeared. And it was not just because we were on holiday with a decent pub within walking distance nor that the weather was being unusually kind.

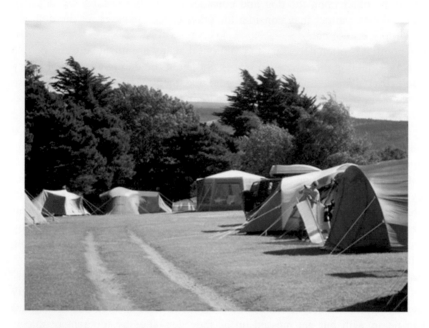

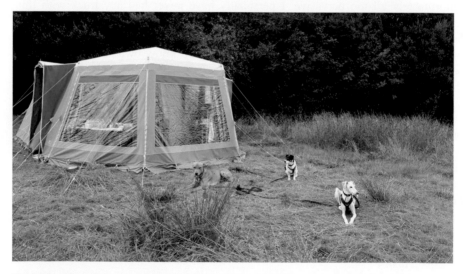

Harmony between dogs and humans when camping!

A grumbling annoyance between us had always been the difference in our individual perceptions of what created safety and security and what was aesthetically pleasing. I was considered to be inviting crime at every turn whereas I thought him an artistic Philistine. I frequently forgot to lock the car or close the windows and to this day may not be able to find a set of keys I was somewhat foolishly entrusted with. He on the other hand saw nothing wrong in fixing the ugliest of padlocks to an otherwise unsecured window frame or shoring up a broken stair spindle with gaffer tape. My apparent lack of concern for security upset him every bit as much as did his obliviousness to what looked nice upset me. So far, so trivial in the grand scheme of things.

But on one such holiday, I suddenly came to the realisation that these causes of domestic discontent simply vanished when camping. Why should this be? The answer was *zips*! Absolutely everything when camping is reliant on the humble zip in all its forms. From sleeping bags to wash bags, sleeping compartments to living quarters, outer tent doors and windows, clothes cases and back packs – doing up zips was an hourly necessity. But in all instances, this action created the appearance of being neat and tidy as well as being secure. Both our needs were therefore fulfilled by the simple action of *doing up zips*. Did it matter that our reasons for doing so differed? Not at all as we were both entirely happy with the result.

Both our *motivations* had been fulfilled by the same *method*.

I subsequently found this experience very useful when counselling the owners of problematic dogs. It helped to avert the intrinsic dangers of playing the blame game. If agreement could be reached about *how* to move forward, even though the reasons *why* differed, harmony could be restored. A little less doting on a dog avoids the routine reward of attention seeking as well as the irritation caused to a disapproving observer. Explaining why ecstatic greetings do not express preferential adoration as assumed does much to quell resentment. Certain aspects of 'tough love' will be needed to emphasise that giving in immediately regarding everything a dog appears to want does not lead to a healthy relationship. This will be approved of by the authoritarian and help to validate their view. Conversely, strongly advising more 'carrot' and less 'stick' to alter the dog's behaviour without coercion will satisfy the view of the softer party.

It is not necessary for parties to be persuaded to agree on *why* they need change as long as they can come to agree about *how* to bring it about. Compromise is always required by both sides.

"By understanding why humans do the things they do and what drives them to change, we can make the world a better place for all animals" is the expressed aim of the HBCA (Human Behaviour Change for Animals) organisation (www. hbcforanimals.com).

In a very small way, Zips Theory may help.

8 The wisdom of children

Some years ago, I visited a family of two adults and four children, the youngest of whom was five years old. They were desperately in need of help with the behaviour of their two-year-old Springer Spaniel who I shall call Sam. He was considered to be the 'naughtiest dog' they'd ever known. When asked to list his various misdemeanours in the pre-consultation questionnaire, after reaching about number ten on the list (which happened to be stealing tea towels), the mother of the family had given up, simply stating that there were 'too many to mention'.

He was also thought to be disobedient, not 'listening' and 'never doing anything he was told'. Going upstairs when told not to was a major crime and when asked how often the dog looked guilty, the answer was 'all the time'.

Pretty much the only thing Sam hadn't done was bite anyone.

After a relatively short time of being in the house, by which time it was becoming abundantly clear that the dog spent much of his day being yelled at, the youngest child piped up, 'You know, Mum, you just can't make him do what he doesn't want to!'

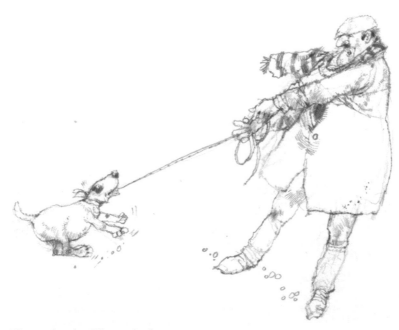

Illustration by Victor Ambrus.

His mother shot him an extremely dirty look. My ill-advised quip that I should leave now and allow the boy to explain his words of wisdom by himself went down

107

like the proverbial lead balloon. But with seemingly precocious understanding, he had hit the behavioural nail on the head.

I have already addressed many of these common misunderstandings elsewhere but the particular interest to me in this case was two-fold.

1. How and why had the young boy appeared to have such accurate insight? How could he see with such clarity what was going wrong in the family's relationship with their dog when his mother appeared ignorant of it?
2. Were some of Sam's actions considered by the family to be 'misdemeanours' for spurious reasons and, as such, were they creating unnecessary conflict?

FIRST ISSUE

Thinking about it afterwards, it occurred to me then that children may suffer from many of the same inconsistencies in response from their parents as dogs do. Many of their decisions as to what to do and how to behave are made on the same basis as for dogs. They may do their homework to stop their parents' crossness and nagging or to avoid missing out on a TV programme they want to watch. They may alternatively force down the cabbage or broccoli as they are promised ice cream afterwards. Or they may simply be children who like doing their homework and eating broccoli, therefore appearing to need no such threats or inducements.

PREMACK'S PRINCIPLE

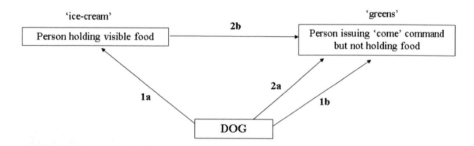

© Kendal Shepherd after Jean Donaldson
2004

PREMACK'S PRINCIPLE

Premack's Principle states that, if a **low probability behaviour** e.g. eating greens, is immediately and reliably followed by a **high probability behaviour** e.g. eating ice-cream, the **frequency** of the low probability behaviour will increase.

'ice-cream'   'greens'

| Person holding visible food | 2b   → | Person issuing 'come' command but not holding food |

1a   2a   1b

DOG

1 <u>Untrained dog</u> The obvious choice of behaviour is to head straight for the person holding food (high probability behaviour) (**1a**) The least obvious choice is to obey the 'come' command, which is so far meaningless, and approach the person with no food in sight (low probability behaviour) (**1b**)

2 <u>Trained dog</u> Low probability behaviour (**2a**) of approaching person saying 'come' but with no food in sight increases in frequency if immediately followed by the approach of the person holding food so dog can eat (**2b**)

In 1965, psychologist David Premack proposed that **a higher probability behaviour can be used to reinforce a less probable behaviour**. He had realised that behaviours themselves could reinforce others and increase their frequency. Premack's Principle is frequently applied in child rearing and dog training. It is also known as relativity theory of reinforcement or "**Grandma's Rule**". The example often given of how high and low probability behaviours interact as they apply to children is eating greens (a low probability behaviour) compared to eating ice cream (a high probability behaviour). The moniker of 'grandma's rule' seems to have been coined owing to the propensity of grandmothers over countless years for making a sweet pudding contingent upon children eating their vegetables first.

What had this child realised about Sam with such percipience and instinct beyond his years? That their dog had to *want* to comply. This was regardless of the reason *why* behavioural decisions were made, or the means whereby outcomes of a chosen behaviour were made clear ('grandma's rule', 'do it or else' or the lure of a lollipop). And so, perhaps without being overtly aware of it, he had experienced these various means of inducing compliance so much himself that he assumed, quite rightly, that the same ought to apply to Sam. Continually attempting to force children or dogs against their will to do something they didn't want to do was on a hiding to nothing.

Some years ago, I recall a media furore resulting from the suggestion, as if it were a new idea, that children who misbehaved in class should be rewarded if their behaviour improved, however marginally. Many complaints arose as a result of the misinterpretation that children were rewarded for being 'naughty' in the first place and that 'good' children were left out. Interesting conversations arising on this subject can still be found on the Mumsnet website from 2008 (https://www.mumsnet.com/Talk/primary/451012-naughty-children-rewarded-for-being-good).

> DD and I were discussing a boy in her class (Y3) who lives round the corner, and she said that he sometimes gets chocolate from Mrs. S (classroom assistant).
> 'Why?' I asked.
> 'Well, it's because he is a naughty boy and if he's good for a week Mrs S gives him chocolate.'
> 'So what do you get for being good all the time, DD?'
> 'Nothing.'
> 'Do you think that's right?'
> **'No!'**

Someone insisted,

> 'Children should not be rewarded for **behaving like everyone else** is expected to behave.'

There was also concern expressed regarding how children could be manipulative and 'work the system', behaving badly then deliberately turning on the charm when necessary to be given rewards.

Alternatively, the question was asked

'Would you insist that only the brightest children get rewarded for academic progress? Would you insist that only those children who are top of the class get stickers? I bet the answer is no. We would all prefer that children should be rewarded for their efforts, regardless of where they are on the academic curve of the class.

'The same is true for behaviour. Do you **only** reward 100% perfect behaviour? Or do you, as an adult, recognise that 'good' behaviour is **harder for some children to attain than others?**'

My Prodigal Son Principle (see Chapter 9 'The educational value of analogy') relates this biblical story and suggests an interpretation relevant to all prodigals, school children and canines included. Rather than being rewarded only for the *best performances*, reward should be given proportional to *difficulty of task* performed. It matters not how long it takes, but once an appropriate, 'good' decision has been made by a miscreant, it must be appreciated and rewarded.

However, we must not forget the child (such as DD in the conversation above) who finds it easy to be good and whose behaviour is at risk of being taken for granted. They perhaps do not need as much encouragement as the naughty child, but we should well understand the perceived unfairness if they are not rewarded at all.

The following anecdote provides an apt example.

Relaxing in a pub garden one sunny lunchtime, I was sitting close to a family consisting of grandmother, mother and two children – a young boy and an even younger girl. I overheard the following exchange. The girl was alternately crying, whining and generally making a fuss. Shortly, the mother went inside to the bar to buy some crisps with the declared intention of 'keeping her quiet' till lunch arrived. As she left, the boy piped up to his grandmother, 'Can I have some crisps as well?' She replied, 'You don't need crisps, dear, because you're being a good boy.'

It was as much as I could do to stop myself jumping up shouting, 'Get him some crisps!'

What is the take-home message from all of this? Are dogs capable of manipulating events on purpose as children might? Although I don't believe they can do it knowingly and deliberately, I accept it can appear so. The owner must be aware of sequences of behaviour becoming linked or 'chained' together. It is often advised to substitute one irritating behaviour, such as jumping up at visitors, with another more convenient one, 'sit to greet' for example. Dogs are perfectly capable of predicting that if they jump up first, they are very likely to be asked to sit immediately afterwards. The 'sit' behaviour then gains a reward. Instead of one behaviour being substituted for another, the danger is that the two behaviours may become linked together. The dog learns to sit, not *in preference* to jumping up, but *jumps up first* in order to be asked to sit. In this way, dogs will appear to be deliberately irritating when in fact they have accidentally been taught to be.

To reward or not to reward? There should be no dilemma. It is of course perfectly possible to appreciate how *difficult* a dog or child finds it to be 'good' and reward accordingly as well as *never taking good behaviour for granted* in either species. The Prodigal Son Principle (Chapter 9 'The educational value of analogy') and the 'Whose idea is it?' rule (Chapter 7 'Avoiding conflict between dog and human') are not mutually exclusive. In this way, dogs and children of all levels of achievement can be appreciated and rewarded appropriately.

SECOND ISSUE

I was also wondering, whether some of Sam's actions were considered to be "misdemeanours" for spurious reasons and, as such, were they creating unnecessary conflict?

On what basis had the misdemeanours of this poor benighted dog been categorised? As simple 'disobedience', or were they supposed transgressions of a more fundamental social nature? Importantly, could the children make sense of it?

It transpired that a considerable amount of parental ire was generated by Sam venturing upstairs, particularly to lie on the bed in one or other of the children's bedrooms. Climbing on the furniture generated a similar response. I questioned why these were considered such major crimes. Not only were they interpreted as evidence of wanton disregard for the owners' instructions, but the owners were also firm believers in the dominance myth and were in imminent danger of passing it on to their children. They were absolutely convinced that if Sam ever got the chance to look down on them from above, he would become bossy and dominant. His disobedience was being taken as evidence that he was already well on the way to assuming his role as leader of the pack.

From then on, it was relatively easy to kill many more than two birds with one stone. I immediately got rid of any notion that being upstairs and above them geographically would have any bearing whatsoever upon his tendency to steal tea towels. Completely unnecessary conflict was being created by their outmoded beliefs. All that was needed was to move Sam voluntarily around the house, including up and down the stairs (otherwise termed 'recall practice'), amply rewarding him all the while. I explained that his irritating behaviours were largely driven by the attention he received when 'misbehaving' and that their efforts to stop him had had the opposite effect to that intended.

Most importantly, I emphasised that the frequency with which he looked 'guilty' (all the time) was a reflection of how often he had been reprimanded, not of how often he knew he'd done something wrong. The reinterpretation of the guilty look, together with an explanation of the gestures on the Ladder of Aggression, really hit home. I made no bones about how lucky they were that Sam had not yet been forced to bite and that this was a testament to his tolerant and forgiving nature.

SUMMARY

1. Sam had to understand exactly what the family wanted him to do, *not* what they didn't want.
2. Shouting what they didn't want ('No!' or 'Stop it!) was not good enough. He (as sometimes the kids) had had to work out by lack of shouting (negative reward) what was required.

3. Unnecessary conflict had been created by the false belief that going upstairs would make Sam 'dominant' and bossy.
4. There had been a potentially dangerous misinterpretation of appeasing and threat averting behaviour as guilt and Sam's acknowledgement of wrongdoing.

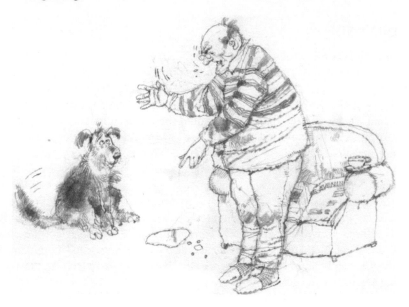

Illustration by Victor Ambrus.

9 The educational value of analogy

This chapter covers
  Analogies to assist in understanding and explaining behavioural principles
  accurately but with no long words!
  The Swimming Pool of Life
  The Prodigal Son Principle
  The Behavioural Iceberg

I am not one for trying to reinvent the wheel under other more fancy names. With respect to dog training and behaviourist colleagues over the years, I do suspect that this is exactly what has happened, to the confusion of all. A new way of describing an age-old truth is dressed up to sound like an invention and called so-and-so's method or rules or even a 'revolution'. The writing was on the wall with *No Bad Dogs: The Woodhouse Way*. Using an amalgam of choke chains, taps on the nose, a commanding voice which brooked no argument and a claimed affinity with animals, her 'way' persuaded many to follow her example and emulate her supposedly unique abilities.

I make no such claims. Having said this, I have found the following analogies extremely useful to explain certain principles in different ways. Hopefully clear and easy to grasp, they are simply reflections of how I myself came to the realisations I did. Take your pick – mark, learn and inwardly digest whichever one you find most useful for you and your clients!

THE SWIMMING POOL OF LIFE

When teaching a child to swim, if we have any sense, we do not throw her into the deep end of the pool and wait to see what happens! If we did, we would find ourselves having to perform emergency rescues on a very regular basis. Instead, we keep the child in the shallow end where they can be taught the motions of swimming while they still have their feet on the ground and therefore feels safe. We then very gradually move towards the deep end, ensuring that the child always knows where the shallow end is and how to reach it. Thus, they never have to panic and they develop confidence in the knowledge of how to 'rescue' themselves.

Yet so often we do not give dogs sufficient (or any) time and opportunity to learn how to cope with situations they find tricky. On a daily basis, dogs find themselves approaching a situation or context they find impossibly difficult to deal with.

113

Because they seem so far outwardly 'fine' (as the child would appear while still on the edge of the pool or standing in the shallow end), nothing is done to intervene with educational guidance. Instead the dog is thrown into a metaphorical deep end. When unwanted behaviour inevitably arises, which illustrates a dog's discomfort and inability to 'swim', it is too often assumed that the dog is being 'difficult' or 'naughty', and he may well be reprimanded. This simply serves to convince the dog that their owner is just as upset by the situation as they are themselves. As such, the owners cannot be relied upon to give guidance and the dog must sink or swim on their own in whatever way they are able.

It is rare for a dog, whose owner has not had the benefit of behavioural advice, to be shown how to follow the steps as one would for a child in a swimming pool. Although this analogy may be applied to a great number of problem contexts, the **behaviour of a dog who is intolerant of other dogs** is a prime example of how a dog may be given inadequate or faulty guidance. Even those who have attended training classes may fall into the trap of trying to tell a dog what *not* to do – to stop barking, lunging and pulling on lead, growling, threatening to bite, etc. – instead of thoroughly teaching what a dog should do *instead of* these unwanted and socially embarrassing actions. Various means are attempted to discourage the dog as well as verbal reprimand, which almost inevitably includes tightening the hold on the lead. The sensation of having no way of escape, heading instead inexorably and un-avoidably towards the 'deep end', is made worse should the lead be connected to a choke chain. Potentially indelible negative associations may thus be made with other dogs.

As with many behaviour 'problems', the solution is to train alternative, more acceptable behaviours by rewarding means. Over time, dogs will come to choose these behaviours for themselves, just as the child who has learned to swim. However, to achieve this, they must be given repeated and consistent information from the owner which predicts rewarding consequences.

We must therefore consider what rewarding consequences will be in this context from a dog's perspective. Although it may appear that the 'misbehaving' dog is intent on battle with another dog, in reality the emotions underlying the behaviour are nearly always fear and anxiety. These emotions are inadvertently made worse by the owner. In other words, attack has become the apparent best means of defence. What such a dog really wants, above all else, is to increase the distance between himself and the other dog and thereby calm both himself and his owner. If restrained on lead and without being shown any other behavioural options, he will attempt to force the other dog to retreat.

The simplest behaviour to train may be the 'sit' while allowing other dogs to pass by, but this alone will not necessarily fulfil all the dog's needs. By slackening the lead, turning *away* from an approaching dog and asking your dog to follow and move 'This way!', three important pressures are brought to bear on his subsequent decision. A dog will risk losing his owner's company as well as the tasty food in their pocket if he doesn't comply (negative punishments). He will also remain in a situation of perceived threat in the form of the approaching dog (positive punishment).

Conversely, if he complies and follows his owner, he will:

a.   regain his owner's company,
b.   be given copious food titbits (both positive rewards), and will
c.   relieve himself of perceived threat and emotional distress by moving *away* from the approaching dog (negative reward).

(For explanation of positive and negative rewards and punishments, see Chapter 4.)

A common mistake is to leave intervention too late. It is *before* a dog reacts, when the dog is still emotionally stable enough to think straight and concentrate, that guidance is required. So often we wait to interrupt a dog's 'bad' behaviour rather than pre-empting it by giving him something else to do. I find that owners are tempted to test out the success of their training efforts by waiting to see if their dog will react. *Never wait and see* what a dog will do! Inevitably, if a dog has already reacted, what we want the dog to do (to pay attention to us) is in opposition to what he now wants (to drive the other dog away). To do what is uppermost in his mind is so at odds with guidance given too late that enormous emotional conflict is created. Attempting to force a dog to obey us does just this.

To reiterate, owners should never wait to see what a dog will do (the equivalent of waiting to see if he can swim in the deep end of the pool) as, by the time the dog has chosen the wrong thing for himself, the owner is very unlikely to be able to change the dog's mind. Both dog and owner will therefore fail. One should always err on the side of caution. Giving guidance early to pre-empt arousal will ensure that what the dog feels he has to do does not outweigh his owner's wishes. It will ensure that his decision is far easier to make and will keep the dog within his depth in his particular pool.

If an owner's pre-emptive guidance is practised calmly and consistently in a light-hearted tone of voice, a dog may begin to anticipate his owner's actions by looking in their direction whenever other dogs come into sight. This shows that they have learned that it is so much more pleasant to follow the owner and stay calm, thus keeping themselves out of the 'deep end' of the pool and in safety.

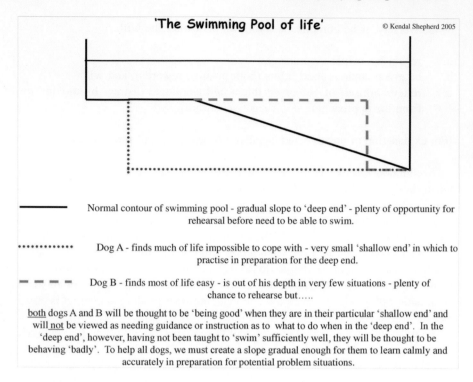

'The Swimming Pool of life' © Kendal Shepherd 2005

Normal contour of swimming pool - gradual slope to 'deep end' - plenty of opportunity for rehearsal before need to be able to swim.

Dog A - finds much of life impossible to cope with - very small 'shallow end' in which to practise in preparation for the deep end.

Dog B - finds most of life easy - is out of his depth in very few situations - plenty of chance to rehearse but.....

both dogs A and B will be thought to be 'being good' when they are in their particular 'shallow end' and will not be viewed as needing guidance or instruction as to what to do when in the 'deep end'. In the 'deep end', however, having not been taught to 'swim' sufficiently well, they will be thought to be behaving 'badly'. To help all dogs, we must create a slope gradual enough for them to learn calmly and accurately in preparation for potential problem situations.

The accompanying diagram illustrates how the dimensions and shape of the swimming pool of life may vary according to the lives and behaviour of individual animals. The normal contour of a swimming pool has a gradual slope towards the deep end and plenty of opportunity to rehearse how to swim before it becomes essential. Two extremes are depicted – **dog A,** who finds much of life very difficult to cope with and therefore has a small shallow end in which to practise, and **dog B,** who misbehaves very rarely with an extensive shallow end.

However, neither dog has a slope provided for them upon which to learn, appearing to be 'good' (behaving well when they can stand) and suddenly 'bad' (as they fall into the deep end).

Procedure of the approach of another dog

- Have especially tasty food treats, which are reserved for difficult situations (cheese, ham, hot dogs) and possibly a squeaky toy for distraction at the ready.
- Allow your dog to curve around another dog rather than force him to approach them head-on or to meet along a pavement. Avoid meeting at narrow entrance or exit gates and give space by, for example, crossing the road or moving off the pavement into a driveway. Create a safety barrier by walking the other side of a parked car (if safe) or by putting yourself as a barrier between the two dogs.
- When you change direction, encourage him to follow you out of choice, using a 'This way!' command and with food treats as lures/rewards rather than pulling him away. Keep the lead as relaxed as possible even to the extent of pretending it is not there.
- Continue to use jolly conversation if it keeps him calm and focused on you.
- If he becomes aroused, do your best not to get cross which will merely increase the threat to him. He is likely to blame the change in you on the other dog rather than on his own behaviour.
- Give him an obedience command, such as 'Watch me!' and 'Sit!' rather than reprimanding him and reward profusely with food and praise if he obeys.
- Do not be tempted to comfort or soothe him after he has become agitated. This risks convincing him that you approve of his behaviour.
- If you have not managed to avoid arousal and he is not listening to your commands, the only non-rewarding option left is to ignore him completely until the other dog has passed by and you feel you can regain his attention. Actively ignore him by standing with your back to him.
- Praise and reward him as soon as he pays you attention again even if you feel tense or upset.

THE PRODIGAL SON PRINCIPLE

There was a wealthy man who had two sons. One, the younger, was dutiful and diligent; the elder, a lazy wastrel. One day, this son, fed up with living under his father's thumb, decided to go out and explore the world. He asked for his share of his inheritance early so he could go out and enjoy himself.

Sometime later, when this money was all spent on wine, women and song, the now destitute young man resolved to return home and beg his father's forgiveness. He would be prepared to earn his keep by looking after his father's herd of pigs to atone for his misdemeanours, if only he was allowed to stay.

Contrary to expectations, his father was overjoyed at his return – so delighted that he ordered three days of partying and festivities to celebrate the occasion. The fatted calf,

reserved specially for such feast days, was to be killed and the whole household to
have a surprise holiday.
The younger son's nose was rather put out of joint by this, somewhat understandably, and
he protested to his father that, in spite of his loyalty and obedience, he had never had so
much as a chicken killed for him and his friends! His father patiently explained that he
received good things every single day and that all the father's remaining wealth would
one day be his. It was therefore quite right that they should celebrate the lost son's return.

Now this biblical tale can be interpreted and told in such a way as to understand and
assist our canine prodigals. My interpretation for this purpose is that the father was
fully appreciative of how almost insurmountably difficult it had been for his son to
come home and apologise. However little the 'bad' son had achieved in his life thus
far was now of no matter. Coming home had been his greatest achievement ever.
The lavish feast had therefore been in due recognition of this achievement.

So how to apply this thought to our canine prodigals?

It is very common to find that a dog's behaviour is compared unfavourably with
that of a companion animal, a neighbour's dog, with that of other dogs in training
class or even one previously owned. And so dogs are labelled and categorised. There
are 'good' dogs who get things right and 'bad' dogs who get it all wrong. We are told
that good dogs deserve reward with the corollary that bad dogs don't.

However, the reality is that when dogs are 'being good', such animals are finding
it easy to make the right decision – in other words, to do things which don't annoy or
upset us. Conversely, dogs behaving badly are finding it impossibly difficult to do the
right thing – in other words, if they have never been shown clearly and meaningfully
what the right thing to do is in the first place. Consequently, good dogs are rewarded
and get even better at being good and bad dogs get nothing. The view often pro-
mulgated in training class is 'they don't deserve it as they haven't earned it'.

The Prodigal Son story tells us differently but may well be counterintuitive.
Reward must be proportional to **difficulty** of the task required, *not* to how **good** the
performance was. One dog should not be compared unfavourably with another but
rewarded amply even for a 'baby step' in the right direction.

Difficulty of task (usually a correct response to an obedience command) must be
considered at all times. A dog may respond on the button when asked to sit in the
kitchen with food on offer, but how about at the vet's or on a walk with rabbits on
the horizon? We must be prepared to recognise difficulty and pay a dog accordingly. At the very moment they may be about to behave the worst, the most must be
on offer as reward if they succeed.

THE BEHAVIOURAL ICEBERG

During a consultation, it is very rare to find that the presenting behavioural
symptom is the only aspect of a patient's repertoire that could do with some considerable tweaking. The presenting problem may well be viewed as the most serious. Behaviours such as barking excessively, escaping from the house and, of
course, having bitten someone can cause considerable inconvenience, anguish and
trauma, not least because the behaviours risk a dog coming to the attention of the

authorities. But it is impossible to treat the problem in hand without taking other, lesser foibles into account. In fact, the perceived lesser misdemeanours may be feeding into the more serious problem, thus acting as the **bulk of a metaphorical iceberg** keeping the tip, the presenting problem, afloat.

The bulk of the iceberg under the water tends to be made up of behaviours which make the owners upset and angry but they have not been considered serious enough to warrant individual attention. They may also have been inadvertently rewarded by the owners giving the irritating behaviours inevitable attention.

Adding to the tip of the iceberg, alongside the presenting problem may be the incidence of concurrent disease (historical disease adding to the underwater bulk). Behaviour may deteriorate owing to the symptoms of the condition itself, particularly if there is any pain or inflammation, and side effects of medication used to treat the condition, for example, corticosteroids, must also be considered.

All contributing factors may be itemised in the accompanying diagram, which can be used to help to focus the mind of clients.

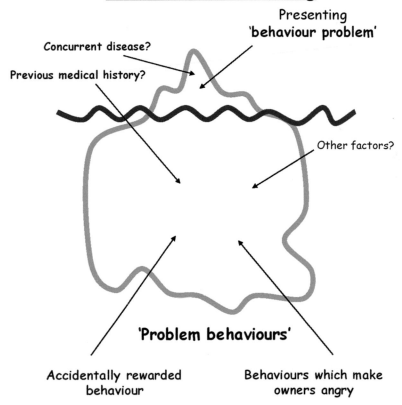

The Behaviour Iceberg

Presenting 'behaviour problem'

Concurrent disease?

Previous medical history?

Other factors?

'Problem behaviours'

Accidentally rewarded behaviour

Behaviours which make owners angry

© Kendal Shepherd 2004

DOODLE'S BEHAVIOURAL ICEBERG

Let me give you the rather extreme example of a little dog called Doodle. It was my encounter with this individual dog that precipitated this concept and the realisation that the owners' initial complaint was merely the tip of a very large iceberg hidden under the water.

Doodle was a 6-year-old neutered male Westie, and his owners had suffered his multiple irritating habits long before he was eventually referred for behavioural help. He had tried to bite an adult visitor and, most concerningly, had bitten one of their young grandchildren. Despite his back story of behaviours which should have been nipped in the bud, the owners thought that these apparently new and alarming events had materialised out of the blue.

As a routine, Doodle barked at the front door and jumped up wildly at visitors and the owners on their return to the house. This had been interpreted as being very pleased to see them and showing off to visitors, and his greeting was returned in kind. He was fearful of thunderstorms during which he was habitually cuddled by the female owner in an attempt to calm him. He used to bark at, chase and sometimes kill hedgehogs and rabbits. Running about willy-nilly in the garden was his main form of exercise when he ignored any attempts by his owners to control him. All these I considered to be behaviours which had been accidentally reinforced with attention of some kind.

On walks, Doodle pulled on lead, showed aggression towards other dogs and had a very poor recall. He also ate the post. These behaviours all made his owner angry whereas his snappiness on being groomed upset them. How could a dog who appeared to greet them so happily also want to bite them?

To conclude his long list of misdemeanours, Doodle became ferocious at the veterinary surgery, particularly in the presence of the female owner, who alternately tried to comfort or became cross with him. Interestingly, this was only mentioned as an afterthought. It seemed far more readily understood, to the extent of being considered more or less normal by the owners, that Doodle should try to bite a vet rather than themselves.

In terms of Doodle's veterinary history, he suffered from Westie-typical skin disease which caused great concern (particularly to his female owner) and had in the past been treated with corticosteroids.

Doodle's Behavioural Iceberg

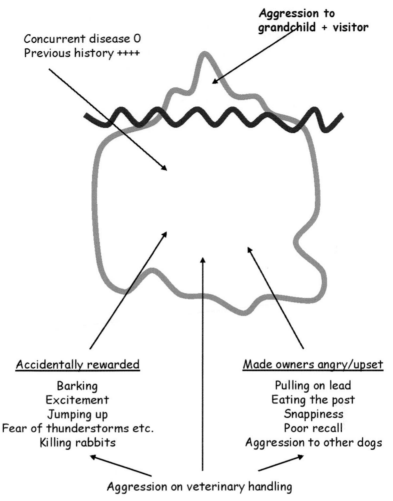

Concurrent disease 0
Previous history ++++

Aggression to
grandchild + visitor

Accidentally rewarded

Barking
Excitement
Jumping up
Fear of thunderstorms etc.
Killing rabbits

Made owners angry/upset

Pulling on lead
Eating the post
Snappiness
Poor recall
Aggression to other dogs

Aggression on veterinary handling

©Kendal Shepherd 2004

In my report, it was first emphasised that it would be impossible to treat Doodles' biting in isolation from the rest of his life. Although the bite to the visitor and their grandson had been precipitated by both the visitors' and grandchild's own behaviour, he was never to be left alone to make his own decisions in the presence of small children in the future. He was also to be kept away from any visitors who had the irresistible desire to say hello and touch him and might be unable to follow future instructions to stay calm and predictable.

What had become abundantly clear was that the owners had only ever made attempts to stop his behaviours. They had not effectively taught him what they would prefer him to do *in advance*.

The advice given was summarised as follows:

1. To rid Doodle of the need to become aggressive, his decision making should be based on anticipation of a positive reward rather than any sense of 'do it or else!' This way he would begin to associate human gestures and commands with pleasure rather than the need to avoid, by whatever means, human anger.
2. The Ladder of Aggression diagram was used to remind them that whatever Doodle had done in the past, including running away, cowering or biting, had all had the intention of calming and dispelling threat. The same mental processes were going on when he rejected attention from his owners by simply walking away or by snapping. They were advised that all their communication with him should produce a raised rather than tucked under tail.
3. Importantly, it had been revealed that food was left down for Doodle to snack at whenever he felt like it. An effective means of manipulating behaviour without entailing threat was therefore being given away for 'free'. Food was to be taken up to prevent him helping himself and thought of as payment rather than an indulgence. They should have the most on offer when he was about to behave the worst, thereby appreciating the *difficulty* he might have in complying.
4. The Scale of Emotion diagram (see Chapter 4) was used to remind them that he would find it easiest to learn when in emotional neutral, in other words, when not chasing rabbits or trying to bite the vet. This was typically when he was 'behaving nicely' and therefore not thought to need any instruction.
5. His greeting behaviour was to be reinterpreted as evidence of stress and as an appeal for calm rather than a request to say hello or be fussed in return. Doodle was plainly threatened by being leant over and touched. Visitors were to ignore him and not touch him under any circumstances, thereby never giving him the opportunity to repel their attentions by aggressive means.

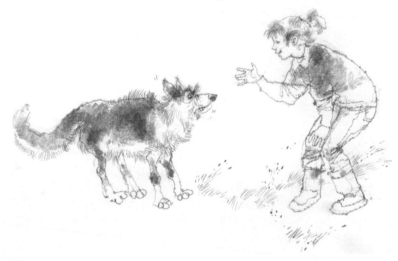

Illustration by Victor Ambrus.

6. His owners were also advised to behave in a more aloof manner towards him and follow the 'whose idea is it?' rule. This would entail using all resources (food, toy, their attention) to reward him if he was calm *of his own volition* or alternatively to use calm times to practise changing his mind. They would also not fall prey to any attention-seeking habits.
7. It was emphasised that letting him out into the garden whenever he wanted was merely giving him the chance to rehearse all the wrong behaviours. They were to 'get his brain in gear' first by asking him to sit before opening the back door and, to begin with, to consider that mental exercise was more important than physical.
8. Above all, they were not to feel mean, guilty or cross.

Finally, it was explained that one couldn't measure progress simply by absence of bites. It was a given that Doodle should have neither the opportunity nor reason to bite again. Improvement in recall, ready interruption of jumping up and barking with a compliant 'come' and 'sit' and increased tolerance of grooming were therefore to be markers of progress.

Although Doodle at the time of the bites was not suffering with his skin, nor under treatment, the associations made in the past between discomfort and veterinary handling were likely to be long-lasting. In addition, if the clock could be turned back, corticosteroids would not have been the treatment of choice. Studies have found that steroids are linked to an increase in nervousness and agitation, as well as, being a 'fight or flight' hormone, enhancing the memory of unpleasant events (Notari and Mills 2016). Attempted comfort or punishment for aggression in this context by his owner had further convinced Doodle that vets were a threat.

CONCLUSION

I have found that each of these analogies is helpful in their own way to illustrate the common difficulties clients face with their pets' behaviour. They highlight in turn frequent mistakes by intervening too late in the sequence of events that leads to 'bad' behaviour (**the Swimming Pool of Life**); that they must consider how hard it will be for their dog to do as they ask and not make unhelpful comparisons with other well-behaved dogs (**the Prodigal Son Principle**); and, finally, that there is no such thing as a minor misdemeanour. All unwanted behaviours that upset us and make us angry or are accidentally rewarded are important and cannot be ignored if thorough diagnosis and treatment is to be attained (**the Behavioural Iceberg**).

10 Walking a mile in a client's moccasins

It is no longer the norm to offer house calls as a routine part of general practice. Pressure of time and money combined, the need to make each minute as profitable as possible, ensuring that every practice has all the toys a new graduate expects (which must then of course earn their keep), the cost of continuing professional development (CPD) now mandatory and enough staff to enable an attractive time-off rota all seem to have conspired to consign the house call to history as an inconvenient and inefficient exercise. Clients are expected to be organised enough to get themselves to the practice and only in an absolute emergency will veterinary staff have to venture out of their comfort zone into the unknown territory of a client's home. Few practices cover their own out-of-hours emergencies, and even then, the travelling must be done by the client to a designated night clinic, often miles from where they live.

There is no doubt that, technically speaking, pet owners are served to a very high standard, but what a wealth of information we may be missing if the environment in which our patients live is largely unknown to us. It would sometimes seem that farm animals have the better deal in this regard. Management systems and environment are routinely considered to have a bearing on their physical health and the incidence of disease and are therefore automatically included in the large animal veterinary surgeon's remit. Not so for the small animal veterinary surgeon and their patients, pet dogs, which may be skidding uncomfortably on a fashionable polished wood floor, subjected to the impact of noise from a multitude of electronic household gadgets or contained and trained with electric shock. Yet their veterinary surgeon may be completely unaware of their plight. How can we truly say such animals are under our care if this is the case?

I may recall with horror the blood and indelible marks of styptic pencil left on what seemed like an acre of pale pink Persian carpet after a home nail clip on a pampered pug went badly awry or the distaste at finding myself in the house of a hoarder, every wall stacked floor to ceiling with newspaper. But such memories are countered by the pride one felt and gratitude received after attending an emergency. My first emergency call-out was to a dog left home alone who had managed to smash its way through a plate-glass window, badly lacerating a leg in the process. As I jumped out of the car, a shopkeeper who happened to recognise me from school days was standing by the stricken animal. He said comfortingly, 'Don't worry, love, the vet's on his way.' With no time to remonstrate regarding gender assumptions, I was more than happy to reply, 'I *am* the vet.'

Information gleaned in home contexts can be invaluable and at least some record should be kept of a client's home circumstances. Vital to the veterinary

125

behaviourist in order to assess environmental impact upon a patient's behaviour, such information should be considered as important to all vets.

INSURANCE

The cost of veterinary attention has, over the course of my career, spiralled out of all proportion, to the extent that few clients, apart from the very well off, can afford the thorough, technologically aided care that can now be provided for their pets. Unless, that is, they are insured. To the benefit of conferences seeking sponsorship as well as dog owners' minds being put at rest, pet insurance has become big business. There may even be a tendency to look upon an uninsured client who finds themselves without the financial wherewithal to afford our excellent services as in some way irresponsible. The lack of financial foresight and planning seems to relegate them to the realms of second-class citizenship. But as with the chicken and egg, which came first?

In this case, I believe the evidence points firmly in the direction of the insurance companies who saw a lucrative niche market to be derived from owners worried about the worst happening to their pet. After all, it was not initially in any general practice's best interests to raise the cost of its services out of the reach of the vast majority of the general public. But with the rise in uptake of insurance policies, specialist vets could afford to splash out on kit which was initially a luxury and then became an essential necessity. Throw media-enhanced client expectations of the miracles that vets could perform into the mix, and the vicious (or virtuous, depending whose side you might be on) circle was complete.

And what of the now ubiquitous corporate practice? It was once anathema to the RCVS to imagine, let alone allow, a veterinary practice to be run by anyone other than veterinary surgeons themselves. Even allowing waiting room sales was un-imaginable, as to do so would seem to lower the profession to the status of mere tradesmen. How times have changed. More and more sole practitioners have been forced to sell their businesses as they find themselves unable to compete with the corporate businesses in terms of attracting employees or keeping clients.

And the consequence? One would have imagined the result to be contented graduates who have everything that their lengthy and expensive education has led them to expect. All the state-of-the-art equipment they need, plenty of time off with no night duties, so as to better enjoy their earnings, and a multitude of grateful clients to add to their immense job satisfaction. I despair when I find that the opposite appears to be true. Unfulfilled vets who think themselves overworked and underpaid and dissatisfied clients believing vets are only 'in it for the money' have become the new norm.

What will help redress the balance? I am of the firm belief that following the principles of behavioural husbandry (see Chapter 2) will create better veterinary surgeons. It will increase day-to-day enjoyment of practice in the knowledge that one has not only enhanced the relationship between the pet and client but also between the pet and the practice as well as improved clinical outcome. How better to create satisfied loyal clients who feel they have been given real value for money at the same time as immeasurably increasing one's own job satisfaction?

I will again show my age when I reveal that, at the time of this illuminating exchange, the basic consultation fee for dogs at the solely small animal practice where I worked was £4.95. it was the practice routine for the consulting veterinary surgeon to inform the client of the financial damage and for payment to be made at reception.

I can't recall what exactly was the problem discussed in the consultation but nothing in the way of medication or investigation needed to be added to the basic fee. There was evident relief on the face of the client as I told her the price. The small boy with her was far more forthcoming and, much to his mother's embarrassment, he piped up immediately, 'That's good! Mum's only got a fiver!'

As I thought about this brief exchange, I realised that, for a child to have come out with such a revealing statement, probably the sole topic of conversation on the way to the surgery if not earlier in the day or all week, was likely to have been their pet, his potential ailments, how serious they might be and, above all, finding out how much it would all cost.

WHO KILLED THE YORKIE?

A recent legal case serves to highlight some of these important issues. On the face of it, when investigating any murder, certainly according to popular TV mysteries, the crime seems initially easy to solve. The cause of death is readily determined and the usual suspects with ample motive and no alibi present themselves. Superficially, the case appears to open and shut with ease.

In this case, a neutered male American cross Japanese Akita I shall call Ronnie escaped from confinement in his garden, crossed that of the immediate neighbour and entered the garden two doors along. He proceeded to pounce upon the resident Yorkshire terrier, Donna, pick her up and shake her, whereupon she went 'limp'. He was fended off with a broom by the Yorkie owner and, being alerted by her screams, his owner retrieved Ronnie and took him home. The Yorkie was taken immediately to a veterinary surgery for treatment but subsequently died. The Akita was taken into custody by the police and the owner of the Akita was charged with the Dangerous Dogs Act Section 3 offence of allowing his dog to be dangerously out of control. So far, so straightforward.

I became involved when instructed by the Akita owner's solicitor to behaviourally assess the dog to give my opinion as to whether he presented any risk or danger to the general public, how obedient he seemed to be and whether any mitigation for his actions could be determined to inform the court's decision as to his fate.

Prior to any behaviour assessment for legal purposes, whenever possible, I ask for the social and medical history of the perpetrator, in this case, Ronnie. I also require the medical history of the victim as it pertains to the incident, whether the victim is human or canine.

Ronnie had been rehomed eight months previously via the breeder, when his previous owner fell ill. He had not been registered with a vet nor had he attended conventional training classes but his owner was 'working on his obedience' at home.

Ronnie could be over-excitable with other dogs and might retaliate if he felt threatened. Play could therefore go badly. Possibly for this reason, he was rarely exercised outside the house but spent most of the time in his back garden. There was no history of aggression towards people. There had, however, been an episode the previous day when Ronnie made his way into the same garden. The properties were owned by the local council and the dividing fences were in a poor state of repair. Although representations had been made to the council regarding the fences and Ronnie's owner had tried to patch his fence up, it was not fully replaced until after the incident and Ronnie had been taken into custody.

When Donna was presented at the veterinary surgery, she was found to have a large flap of skin torn away from her lateral chest wall. There was no record of other injuries, neither of any investigation (in the form of radiography or ultrasound) to eliminate internal injury. She was given intravenous fluids and anaesthetised in order to repair the tear. She was kept in overnight, ate a little the next morning and, presumably as she seemed well enough, was discharged with oral antibiotics to be re-examined in three days' time.

At this post-operative examination, the skin flap was found to have lost its blood supply and had become necrotic, in effect had died. Enquiries were made about referring her to an unnamed specialist unit, following which a quote of between £8,000 and £10,000 was given for the cost of the treatment of such an injury. Not surprisingly, this was way beyond the means of the owner of an uninsured dog living in a council house. The general practitioner therefore proceeded to debride the necrotic skin himself, resuture the remaining skin and a body wrap was applied. The dog was sent home the same day as again she ate a little but was found dead by her owner the next morning.

No post mortem examination was performed but the putative cause of death was described on the records as 'overwhelming infection'.

My assessment of Ronnie, carried out after some six months' in police custody, showed him to be of excellent temperament, affectionate and tolerant of all provocations (including veterinary examination) that the assessment, of necessity, entailed. By this time, the police officer in charge of the case had 'fallen in love' with him. He also showed a good level of obedience, responding readily to the 'sit', down', 'give paw' and 'on your bed' instructions in exchange for food. When confined in a cage, he became aroused at the sight of a Jack Russell brought into view, but if outside the cage, and wearing a head collar for security, he was far calmer and continued to respond to commands when in her close presence. He showed no aggression throughout.

The decision of the court was that his owner was not 'fit and proper' as required by the law (see Chapter 12) and Ronnie was not allowed to be returned to him. My conclusion, taking all information, including my assessment, into account, was that he presented no risk to the public and that he should be allowed to be rehomed to a suitably experienced and responsible owner. I expressed my opinion that the incident itself, although superficially the result of inadequate fencing, was more fundamentally owing to the complete lack of owner appreciation of the effects of social frustration upon his dog. Ronnie's inept social behaviour towards other dogs had led, as is so often the case, to restriction and social isolation, with the inevitable result of emotional frustration, lack of self-control and behavioural deterioration. I also felt that the emotional reward of his escape the day before had reinforced and led to repetition of the behavioural means of this success.

With no dispute as to the identity of the perpetrator or owner and a dead victim, on the face of it surely this was an open and shut case. Or was it?

WHY DID THE YORKIE DIE?

It goes without saying that, had Ronnie not been left on his own outside, or his owner had ensured that the fence was secure, he could not have escaped and Donna would still be alive. Ideally, behavioural advice and steps should have been taken early in the new ownership to allow Ronnie to be exercised safely in the presence of other dogs. But we can all be wise in hindsight. The law, strictly applied, needs only a victim (in this case, unlike many others, entirely blameless) and an admitted perpetrator, for a case to be made out. Ronnie's actions resulted in the Yorkie's demise for sure, but what other factors were involved?

I cannot help but be left with the feeling that the unfortunate Donna and her owner were poorly served by the veterinary community. She appears to have fallen between two stools – those of inadequate care on one hand and no doubt excellent but exorbitantly expensive care on the other. Given the cause of the injury, surely a minimum of an x-ray to eliminate internal damage would have been advised? A post mortem examination was not carried out. (I don't think I am being overly cynical to suggest that this omission was possibly to avoid the risk of hitherto undiagnosed damage being discovered.) A diagnosis of overwhelming infection was given with no material evidence to back it up. These would be considered parlous omissions, to be pounced on by the defence, even if this were a fictitious murder enquiry.

If nothing else, this tale should alert those in general practice that if there is even the remotest possibility of legal consequences, meticulous records should be kept of all procedures. The reasons why they were not carried out, although advised, are as important as detailing what was done. An accurate cause of death must be given with evidence that supports it. If not, courts are left with the inevitable default image of a savage dog tearing its hapless victim limb from limb.

As to the cost of up to £10,000 being given as a quote over the telephone without examining the dog in question, I am pretty much speechless. Have specialist units become so used to rectifying the results of general practice ineptitude and seeing insured patients or those belonging to the well-off only that they can charge what they like? I understand that all procedures have an attendant cost which has to be covered but question the ethics of further distressing an already traumatised client by asking her to make what turned out to be a life-or-death decision on the basis of such huge expense.

Ronnie was subsequently allowed to be released and rehomed via an Akita rescue organisation. All the contributory factors to his escape as well as to the Yorkie's death were included in the report for the court. Without such mitigation being presented on his behalf, it is without doubt that an essentially extremely good natured but mismanaged animal would have been destroyed.

CONCLUSION

It may seem that the opinions I have expressed in this chapter are simply those of an elderly vet harking back to the good old days. But it pains me to read of young vets suffering with stress-related mental health issues and changes of career being forced on them by dissatisfaction with the veterinary profession. I will consider myself a vet until my dying day and know that the knowledge and insight I have accumulated about the behaviour of canine patients have vastly enhanced the enjoyment of general practice. I can only hope that this book will serve the same purpose to others.

Part III

Dogs and the law

Part III

Dogs and the law

11 Vets and the law

> **This chapter covers**
> Overview of UK Dangerous Dogs legislation
> Injustices and inadequacies of the Dangerous Dogs Act
> Behaviour assessment of 'dangerous' dogs
> Implications of neutering and euthanasia
> Need for universal preventative education regarding canine aggression
> Veterinary responsibility under the Animal Welfare Act

This chapter is not intended to be a comprehensive overview of all law pertaining to dogs. It will concentrate on two pieces of legislation of greatest relevance to the veterinary surgeon in general practice – namely, the Dangerous Dogs Act and the Animal Welfare Act. It will highlight the responsibility placed upon veterinary surgeons if the law and its implications are taken seriously. For a summary of all dog law, *A Practical Guide to Dog Law for Dog Owners and Others* by lawyer Andrea Pitt provides useful information. The chapter will also address the issue of behavioural assessment of allegedly dangerous dogs and how care must be taken by all those involved to ensure that such assessments are valid, informative and welfare oriented.

THE DANGEROUS DOGS ACT 1991

This section comprises an overview of this specific legislation, liberally sprinkled with a personal view of its injustices and inadequacies. Although there is other, much older legislation that deals with out-of-control dogs, namely the Dogs Act 1871, this civil law is far less commonly used and will not be discussed here. The vast majority of cases in which I have been involved are brought under the more recent Dangerous Dogs Act 1991, under which both civil and criminal charges may be brought.

The sections of the UK Dangerous Dogs Act (DDA) of most relevance are Sections 1, 3 and 4b. Sections 1 and 3 are both **criminal offences** whereas Section 4b is **civil**. Section 3 applies to dogs of any breed, deemed dangerous because of **what they have done** whereas Sections 1 and 4b apply to dogs deemed dangerous purely **by appearance**, so-called breed-specific legislation or **BSL**. An owner whose dog is of a breed automatically labelled dangerous, and in addition has done something deemed dangerous, will be charged under both Sections 1 and 3 of the Act. Section 4b is reserved for owners of dogs who have not behaved dangerously but are thought to be dangerous by appearance. All dogs thought to look dangerous are mandatorily seized by the police and taken into custody, apart from those dogs and their owners deemed eligible for the Interim Exemption Scheme (IES). Introduced in 2015, the IES allows friendly, non-aggressive dogs, if owned by law-abiding citizens, to remain at home under certain conditions prior to cases coming to court. Not all police forces use this scheme to date; notably, the Metropolitan Police do not.

There is discretion regarding the seizure of dogs which have behaved dangerously. If allowed to remain at home, an interim control order may be made to minimise risk. If the risk of 'recurrence' is thought to be too great, a dog will be seized to 'protect the safety of the public'. Such seizure may, however, not occur for some time after the incident itself.

The main financial and practical significance to any dog owner falling foul of this law is that, if charged under 4b, the civil offence, **legal aid is unavailable**. Legal aid is only available for criminal offences, i.e., if charged under Sections 1 and/or 3. The practical result is that if charged under 4b, defendants have to foot the bill of any legal action themselves or find other means of financial support. However much they believe their dog not to be of a banned breed or type, they may simply be unable to afford the cost of mounting a defence.

Sections 1 and 4b of the Act apply to four dogs – the Pitbull terrier, Japanese Tosa, Dogo Argentino and Fila Braziliero, the proscribed breeds. All considered under the law to be fundamentally 'fighting dogs', it is illegal to own, breed from, sell or give away any such animal. The only dog which does not have a UK-recognised breed standard by which to be identified is the Pitbull terrier. However, this is the only 'breed' of any significance in this country, only a handful of the other breeds ever being found in the UK. In 1993 when it was realised that breed identification was problematic, to say the least, case law determined that the 'type' of dog should be considered instead of breed. As no breed standard for the Pitbull terrier exists in the UK, the American Dog Breeders Association (ADBA) standard, as created in 1974, was selected as the yardstick by which any dog suspected of being a Pitbull type was to be assessed.

Initially when the law was passed, and the owner was found guilty of this crime, it was mandatory for the dog to be destroyed. But in 1997, the law was amended to allow such dogs to be entered onto an Exempt Register providing certain conditions were met. Conditional Destruction Orders were introduced, the conditions of which included that the dog must be permanently identifiable (initially by tattoo, now by microchip), kept muzzled and on lead at all times in public, neutered and insured for third-party liability. Any contravention of these conditions could result in the dog's destruction.

These conditions were all thought to contribute to public safety. Furthermore, the owner had to be considered a 'fit and proper' person and the dog itself had to be shown 'not to constitute a danger' to the general public. The fact that only human-friendly, non-aggressive dogs are allowed onto a register for dogs deemed automatically dangerous by breed type and conformation is a supreme irony.

If the owner is thought unsuitable or not fit and proper, the dog can only be given into the care of a person who is already familiar with the dog. They may then apply to become the **registered keeper** of the dog although ownership does not change. If no such person is found, however good and 'non-dangerous' the temperament of the dog, it must be destroyed.

In addition to these caveats and restrictions, Sections 1 and 4b of the DDA unusually carry a reverse burden of proof: in other words, the defendant is guilty until proved innocent, in contrast to almost all other legislation. The onus is therefore on the defendant to prove his dog is not of the type, rather than on the prosecution to prove it is. The standard of proof is, however, less than other cases. Instead of a case having to be proved beyond reasonable doubt, the lesser burden of proof, *on balance of probabilities*, is supposed to lessen the onus on the defendant. In practise, however, and perhaps cynically I have found the opposite to be true. 'On balance of probabilities' seems to be interpreted rather along the lines of 'no smoke without fire'. If there is some doubt that the dog is of type, yet a charge of owning a Pitbull has been brought by the authorities (the 'smoke'), then it is assumed that a 'fire' must exist and the dog in question 'probably' is indeed a Pitbull type.

Determining type rather than breed has resulted in almost any short-coated, well-muscled mongrel dog being at risk of being labelled a Pitbull by the over-zealous authorities, particularly if in the hands of a person who has already come to their attention for other reasons and is deemed 'dodgy'. As previously stated, whether the dog has behaved in a dangerous manner is immaterial. Staffordshire Bull terriers and crosses thereof are the most likely to be caught up in the net, but even purebred American Bulldogs and crosses of Weimeraners, Neapolitan mastiffs, Dogges de Bordeaux, Rhodesian Ridgebacks (even with ridge!) and Boxers have all been identified by the police as Pitbulls. Type, like beauty, would appear to be in the somewhat prejudiced eye of the beholder.

This indiscriminate inaccuracy is compounded by the reverse burden of proof, which means that no evidence whatsoever has to be routinely provided by the prosecution to the court as to why a police Dog Legislation Officer considers a particular dog to fall into the category of 'type known as the Pitbull terrier'. 'If I say it is, then it is!' is more or less the assertion by seizing officers, and courts are duly guided by a single sentence in an officer's statement to this effect in order to pronounce guilt. In addition, owners may be put under a great deal of pressure to forgo any attempt to disagree with these 'experts'. The 'carrot' of having their dog returned to them in a matter of weeks, rather than months, if not years, provides irresistible emotional persuasion to give in and admit 'guilt' in order to get their dog home as quickly as possible, even with completely unnecessary restrictions.

The upshot is that the vast majority of dogs are entered onto the Exempt Register without any second opinion or accurate determination of the degree to which a dog conforms to the ADBA breed standard. There is also no recognition of how many characteristics of certain 'non-dangerous' breeds may be shared.[1] This is despite the rather nebulous and circular case law caveat stating the following:

---

[1] The result has been what can be described as a form of visual 'Chinese Whispers', in which the myth of what composes a Pitbull is ever enlarged and distorted.

There is an absence of any precise criteria by which a pit bull terrier may be identified positively as a breed and by this means distinguished from all other dogs. One must of course be careful not to extend the application of this section to dogs which are not described in it. A dog must be of the type known as a pit bull terrier if the section (of the Act) is to be applied to it. (cited in R v Crown Court at Knightsbridge ex parte Dunne and Brock 1993)

Those owners who are sure that the police have got it wrong may seek a second opinion but, particularly if self-funding, it is very much an uphill struggle for them as affording a defence often proves impossible. Without the financial means to engage legal representation, they have no way to oppose the police view and are forced to plead guilty by default.

Yet the number of these mongrel dogs entered onto the Exempt Register by these, at best, questionable means is used as evidence of the law's success. To date, the government has been persuaded by the powers-that-be that the law must remain unchanged as it has supposedly cleared the streets of so many 'dangerous' animals.

AND WHAT OF THE FACTS?

From 2007 to 2018, I personally assessed 198 dogs all alleged to be Pitbull types, bearing in mind that these cases only represented owners who had both the temerity and the necessary financial wherewithal to disagree with the opinion of the police. Of these 198 dogs, 26 of them (13%) had also done something the law defined as 'dangerous', namely, the nebulously termed condition of being 'dangerously out of control'. (Ironically, as stated above, the owners of these 26 dogs which had actually done something dangerous and therefore had also been charged under Section 3 of the Act were eligible for legal aid.) Of these 26 dogs, in all cases, people were bitten: eight while ill-advisedly intervening during dog-on-dog incidents, five cases were as a result of owner conflict with the police while resisting arrest, three cases featured groups fighting with each other in the street and two 'domestics'. The remaining few cases similarly reflected human rather than canine failing – an owner drunk in charge of his dog who ran off and nipped playing children, a dog left unattended outside a shop (the proverbial accident waiting to happen) and a 'victim' kicking an approaching off-lead dog in panic.

Of the total of 198 dogs, I assessed only four dogs as truly dangerous in that there was real risk of them biting again. Apart from the finding during the assessment that the dogs needed little discernible provocation to display aggression, given their past history, the bites inflicted were likely to be very serious, even in the most capable hands. I therefore recommended euthanasia for these four.

WHAT OF CASES UNDER SECTION 3 OF THE ACT?

This applies to any dog that has done a 'dangerous' thing and, as such, the owner is charged with allowing the dog to become 'dangerously out of control'. In other words, being 'dangerously out of control' is defined as a dog that has injured or put someone in fear of injury. (Charges arising simply because a potential victim was frightened by a dog are much less common as a case is harder to prove. An injury, on the other hand, speaks for itself.) To put the circular definition the other way round, if a dog injures, it is assumed to have been dangerously out of control at the time, however brief the moment in time happened to be. Even a dog on lead and sitting by his owner's side just prior to biting may be deemed 'dangerously **out** of control', a fact of which few owners are aware. Standard physical control methods alone are not enough to ensure lack of danger, either in the eyes of the law or in reality.

Of course, 'behaving dangerously', as defined by what transpired in one moment in time, is not the same as 'being dangerous' *per se* any more than losing one's temper on occasion is evidence of psychopathology. While they may well accept that their dog has bitten, many owners quite understandably baulk at the assumption that their dog is dangerous. I have found a complete cross-section of breeds involved over the last 20 years and, although the Staffordshire Bullterrier seems over-represented, this may be simply a reflection of its present popularity and the density of the breed and crosses thereof in certain areas of the country. Out of 144 cases, more than one-third of offences arose from dog-on-dog incidents. Although the true target of a dog's aggressive intent had been another dog, aggression was redirected towards a person. Social frustration between dogs appears to be a major cause of inadvertent bites and other injuries to people, including the dog's owner themselves. One does wonder whether measures imposed and taken in attempts to keep people safe, such as restricting the freedom of dogs, have backfired and inadvertently created more antisocial canine behaviour. Owners may also have become more cautious and overly protective of their dogs in view of the threat implicit in the legislation.

In other cases, as under Section 1, 'bad' human behaviour in terms of violence and alcohol consumption featured strongly as well as complete lack of awareness of the stressful and alarming effect unpredictable human behaviour, particularly that of children, can have on dogs. It has become abundantly clear that dog bite incidents are largely unforeseen events, by either owner or victim, and that punishing a misdemeanour after the event alone, with no education as to what led to the bite or its prevention, is doomed to failure.

Although the number of dog bites overall seemed to be rising rather than falling as intended, in the dubious wisdom of those in charge, a law that was spectacularly ineffective in public was in 2014 also applied to private places. Consequently, all the mistakes that were being made in public now could result in an offence being committed on private property as well. As could have been predicted, similar (at best misguided and at worst appalling) human behaviour was evident in dog bite cases occurring at home. Drunken rows, thrown food, girlfriend accusing boyfriend of 'commanding' a dog to attack her, children attempting to pick up or otherwise disturb sleeping dogs, even, on one occasion, putting a basket over a dog's head to 'protect' it from a thunderstorm, all resulted in 'dangerous dog' allegations. **As in public, dogs pushed beyond the limits of social endurance have been forced to bite by an onslaught of ignorance.**

Consequently, prosecutions and convictions of dog owners rose and were heralded as evidence of an effective law. Yet as with Section 1 of the act, Section 3 is fatally flawed.

Firstly, the offence of allowing a dog to be 'dangerously out of control' is, like speeding, a **strict liability** offence and, apart from rare cases where the identity of the canine culprit is in doubt, a guilty plea is mandatory. At least if there is a risk of driving too fast, drivers are given clues as to *how to avoid* offending by way of speedometers in their cars and roadside warning signs. There is no such equivalent knowledge made clear to prevent a dog biting, and the owner is charged out of hand.

Finding someone who can be conveniently *blamed* for allowing their dog to bite does not equate to identifying *cause*, the reason why the bite occurred. Only by identifying cause and using this information in a pre-emptive and educational manner will there be much hope of a reduction in incidence of dog bites. I made a suggestion as to how the problem could be redressed by likening current speed awareness workshops with proposed courses giving vital information regarding dog behaviour (Shepherd 2013). They could be offered in the same way, the reward for attendance being the avoidance of further punishment. As with speeding, there are very common causes and contributory factors to dog bite incidents. Highlighting these should serve to alert dog owners to the conditions and events that led up to a so-called unpredicted dog bite incident and enable avoidance of reoffence.

Secondly, **provocation is not permissible** as a defence under UK law. If thoroughly investigated and analysed from the dog's perspective, mitigation for the dog's actions can be brought, stressing all the while how fundamental ignorance on the part of both 'victim' and dog owner is a major contributary factor. Such mitigation may be sufficient to reduce a sentence to the minimum, but a guilty plea is mandatory all the same.

The result of the strict liability nature of the law has been the fact that dog bite incidents have never, in the history of the DDA, been investigated properly by the authorities, as they should be if it were any other crime. In the normal way, evidence would have to be brought to court to prove the case. As it is, if the identity of the perpetrator is undisputed and 'the dog did it' is sufficient to secure a conviction, another proverbial open and shut case goes down in history. Add this to the fact that provocation is not allowed as a defence, there has never been any onus or *responsibility imposed upon people* to behave sensibly and respectfully around dogs. The fact that certain breeds have been designated as dangerous has created the unforeseen assumption among the public, dog owning or not, that other breeds are safe. The law in all its aspects has created a false sense of security.

The ramifications of all these legal imperfections are far reaching. Common criticism levelled at the breed-specific aspects of dangerous dog legislation concludes that it is unjust, illogical, inhumane and, above all, in no way fulfils the original purpose of the law, namely that of dog bite prevention. Breed Specific Legislation has been roundly condemned by high-profile organisations and the general public alike. In particular, the RSPCA's thoroughly researched report on Breed Specific Legislation published in 2016, aptly named 'A Dog's Dinner' (www.rspca.org), added well-argued weight to their 'End BSL' campaign.

In addition, the Environment, Food and Rural Affairs (EFRA) Committee conducted an enquiry in 2017 into the whole issue of 'dangerous dogs' and the efficacy of legislation. The enquiry was conducted under the auspices of Neil Parish MP, and its report was published in September 2018. The conclusions reached included that the current legislative approach was thoroughly ineffective and that urgent changes were indicated to avoid needless dog deaths. The report strongly recommended comprehensive public education regarding the nature and cause of canine aggression. Despite these conclusions, no change to the legislation has occurred at the time of writing and the government response to this report was generally disappointing. It did, however, provide some light at the end of the legal tunnel. Among recommendations made were that the 'Government should commission an independent review of the effectiveness of the Dangerous Dogs Act 1991 and wider dog control legislation.' Also there should be carried out a 'comprehensive independent evidence review into the factors behind canine aggression, the determinants of risk, and whether the banned breeds pose an inherently greater threat'.

This is currently being undertaken by Angus Nurse, Associate Professor of Criminology and Sociology at Middlesex University.

Both the EFRA report and government response to it can be found here in PDF form:

https://www.parliament.uk/business/committees/committees-a-z/commons-select/
environment-food-and-rural-affairs-committee/inquiries/parliament-2017/dangerous-
dogs- breed-specific-legislation--17–19/

Universal humane education from primary school upwards regarding the nature of dogs and the dog-human relationship is vital if dog bites are to be prevented. Dog bite incidents are invariably described as 'attacks', thus completely prejudicing the public view, including that of magistrates and judges and police, as to a dog's motives. They are dog bite *incidents*, no more and no less. Bites do not come out of the blue: we create them. Human behaviour change is of the essence.

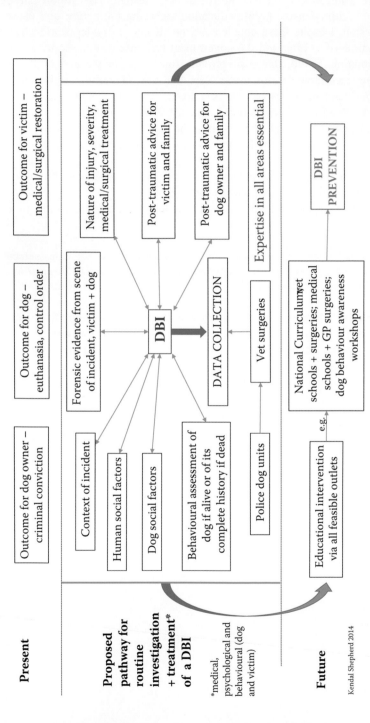

Author's suggestion for the thorough investigation of dog bite incidents to enable universal education as published in RSPCA 'Breed Specific legislation - a dog's dinner' report 2016'.

BEHAVIOURALLY ASSESSING 'DANGEROUS' DOGS

Dogs may be seized under both sections of the Act. Dogs alleged to be Pitbull types are mandatorily taken into police custody (unless allowed to remain at home under the IES, see page 134) despite lack of evidence that they have behaved, or are behaving, dangerously. Under Section 3, dogs which have been 'dangerously out of control' and caused injury are generally seized. Slightly worrying, if a dog really does present a danger, is the fact that the seizure itself, carried out in order to 'protect' the public, may not take place until several weeks after the incident itself.

A behavioural assessment is requested to gauge, as far as possible under artificial conditions, whether a particular dog, if released, will present a danger to the public in real life. The conclusions must include any measures that one feels necessary to ensure safety. Standard measures include keeping a dog on lead and muzzled in public places, and a control order to this effect may be made. However, these physical restrictions are often the only measures relied upon by the courts to prevent future mishap. Common sense dictates that if the primary cause of an incident is a dog escaping from the house or garden, then ensuring the gate is dog-proof and routinely kept securely closed is vital. Dogs do not put on their own muzzles before making a bid for freedom.

A behavioural assessment of an allegedly dangerous dog, in a nutshell, is a simply a means of **diagnosing cause** of any incident and creating an accurate as possible **prognosis** for the future. As with physical disease, when symptoms and their duration are essential for accurate diagnosis, this process must entail gathering as much information about the incident as possible. This information is obtained initially from witness statements, including that of the victim or complainant, hospital records giving details of any injuries and the history of the dog from the owners as well as from the dog's registered veterinary practice.

In an ideal world for seized dogs, records of how the dog has behaved while in custody and how he has been managed should also be routinely available. Unfortunately, one is often left with the suspicion that the worse a dog's behaviour in kennels is, the better it serves to justify seizure and to 'prove' the prosecution's case. A dog and its behaviour are 'bagged and stored' as any other evidence. Well-meaning kennel staff may be instructed not to interact with certain dogs to ensure the detainee does not appear 'nicer' than it should. Several years ago, I had the pleasure of assessing a dog called Stella Hastie, an alleged Pitbull supposedly too 'dangerous' to handle, who had been kept without exercise and little human interaction for two years. The brave actions of kennel staff whistle-blowers who risked their jobs by disobeying police instructions ensured that her case hit the public eye (https://www.bbc.co.uk/news/uk-england-devon-35635935).

As far as I am concerned, the dog's initial behaviour on seizure should be video recorded as evidence of 'danger'. Thereafter, every effort should be made to make the dog's confinement more bearable and to ensure as far as possible that the requirements of the Animal Welfare Act are adhered to. As it is, the requirements of the Dangerous Dogs Act seem to routinely contravene those of the Animal Welfare Act. A conundrum indeed.

In human terms, it is now a legal requirement for 'Independent Custody Visiting' to be allowed for all those held in detention, whatever their crime. Access to detainees must be allowed at any time so that spot checks can be carried out as to their condition and welfare (see the Independent Custody Visiting Association website https://icva.org.uk/). Whether the conditions of detention and a detainee's mental state might affect their fitness to be interviewed is also taken into account. How dogs are cared for and their welfare would be vastly improved if such a system were mandatory for those dogs in police custody. Moves are afoot to introduce such a scheme with the support of representatives of the RSPCA along the lines of the Police Dog Welfare Scheme which has been introduced in various forces following the death of a police dog during training. (see for example https://www.cheshire-pcc.gov.uk/get-involved/volunteering/police-dog-welfare/)

In my experience, assessors carrying out behavioural assessments for the defence are not allowed into the holding kennels unless the dogs are deemed too dangerous to be transported elsewhere. Many of these dogs have been kennelled for many months and could well be aggressive towards strangers. These encounters taught me that nothing could possibly be achieved if I set out to get the dog to do only what I wanted it to do. Of vital importance is to consider what information such dogs need from the assessor, as well as what information the assessor needs from the dogs.

It would seem that some assessors think it valid to provoke the subject in various ways with increasing intensity to ascertain their level of tolerance and at what point the 'straw breaks the camel's back'. In other words, it is the assessor's perceived needs only which drive the contents of the assessment, rather than those of the dog. Although there is indeed an obligation to analyse and rationalise a previous incident, there is no need to force history to repeat itself in order to achieve this and to create a prognosis. By using the medical equivalent, it becomes obvious that we do not diagnose a disease condition by trialling what treatment makes it worse but by what approach results in an improvement. The same is true for behaviour. Determination of the dog's character, preferences and triggers to explain the past and how behaviour can be changed for the better in the future is of the essence.

If a dog has been left at home, one often has the advantage of being able to visit the site of the incident and replicate or verify aspects of it, such as how likely the dog is to have jumped up or chased a passer-by, or how far it ran before an alleged bite was inflicted. It is not unusual for the witness statements to conflict with each other and for a 'victim', possibly for understandable reasons, to assert that the dog ran further or bit more often than is actually the case. Indeed, if detailed medical records can be obtained, including photographs, the injury may not be identified as a dog bite at all, but instead as scratches inflicted by a dog's claws or the result of the victim tripping and falling. As the law applies to injuries 'however caused', not just by a bite, the dog cannot be exonerated by this fact and an owner must plead or be found guilty. Of course, whether the dog was motivated to bite or not and whether the episode was instead the result of victim panic makes a great deal of difference to one's behavioural conclusions.

One is also able to see first-hand how a dog behaves towards strangers knocking on the door, entering the home and greeting the dog in possibly ill-advised but very common ways. A more realistic picture of a dog's behaviour (for better or worse) may then be ascertained compared to the response of a dog confined on its own for a number of months in kennels. Other everyday experiences and responses can be tested in both contexts, such as propensity for food guarding or undergoing veterinary examination. However, one must be aware of the risk of creating false positive as well as false negative responses. A dog may see no reason to guard food when on its own in police kennels but become mountainous in defence of a food bowl in its own kitchen with the owners, their children and a companion dog in close proximity. As is common in the veterinary context, the presence or absence of the owner during examination can make all the difference to a dog's response, again for better or worse.

> Anecdotal evidence gathered via Veterinary Voices private discussion Facebook page during the Covid19 outbreak, when dogs had of necessity to be taken from their owners for veterinary examination, points strongly towards dogs being less stressed and better behaved in their absence. Comments made as to the reasons why included that the lack of the inevitable human social interaction that would occur if the client were present allowed for such examinations to be carried out with sole focus on the dog in question, in particular on its individual behavioural needs. It may be worth bearing these very valid suggestions in mind as to why dogs were almost without exception more content, when veterinary life returns to 'normal'. ('Owner-absent examinations' https://www.vettimes.co.uk/articles/kendal-shepherd/)

In summary, enough should be done within safety limits to form as accurate as possible all-round view of a dog's temperament, personality and behavioural proclivities. Great care, however, must be taken that the means of ensuring safety in an assessment do not falsely indicate the very behaviour the law is intended to prevent (for example, by unessessarily muzzling or tethering a dog) – hence the need for a thorough behavioural history from the owners prior to an assessment. Sometimes it seems that assessors are overly cautious and unnecessarily misled, as are the general public, into imagining that on the basis of one context-specific incident alone, a dog may become savage at any time. It is also of the utmost importance to be entirely unbiased, as is one's sworn obligation, and not be tempted or persuaded either to paint a rosier or more damning picture of a dog than is the case. An identical report should be able to be written to inform the court regardless of whether one is instructed by the prosecution or defence.

For more detailed information on assessing dogs for the courts, see K. Shepherd, 'The assessment of dogs for legal cases – a UK perspective' in *Dog Bites: A Multidisciplinary Perspective*, editors Daniel Mills and Carri Westgarth (2017).

VETERINARY RESPONSIBILITY REGARDING NEUTERING AND EUTHANASIA

Neutering is mandatory for dogs found to be a banned breed and a necessary condition for a dog to be allowed entry onto the Exempt Register. It is still thought by many to be a means of automatically reducing aggression and generally improving behaviour despite evidence to the contrary. Particularly if castration is carried out at or around puberty, the sudden removal of testosterone in young dogs may result in an increase in fear-related aggression (McGreavy 2018). As both sexes may display an increase in aggressive tendencies, the beneficial effect of surgical intervention alone should not be assumed (see Overall 2007 for a review of the literature regarding neutering of bitches). The history and nature of any dog ought to be taken into account before any irreversible procedure is carried out, whether or not the dog is subject to legal proceedings.

Was the cause of an incident related in any way to a dog's hormonal status? As far as possible, dogs in police custody should be treated as any other dog presented to the veterinary surgery for neutering of either sex. A full behavioural history should be taken *before* surgery so that, at least, the owners can be fully informed regarding potential post-operative fallout. Yet it is frequently assumed that the owners of seized dogs have no say in the matter, and consequently a history is not sought, let alone acted upon. A court order has been made that stipulates neutering as a condition of release which makes it imperative for neutering to be carried out. Why worry whether neutered dogs are considered 'safer'? What does an owner (or in the case of the Dangerous Dogs Act, society) expect the result should be, and will neutering live up to expectations? Neutering will quite possibly contribute to the creation of a false sense of security around such dogs.

Behavioural intervention is essential to ameliorate any potential deterioration following surgery as well as to address the issues that led to a 'dangerous' incident in the first place. Behaviour work should also reduce risk, should inevitable human failing recur, by, for example, improving recall. But unfortunately, customary physical impositions are made without taking any behavioural analysis or implications into consideration. Indeed, any behavioural intervention can only be 'strongly advised' by the courts, not made obligatory. Educating all parties – dog, dog owner and 'victim' – is of primary importance if dog bite incidents are to be prevented.

Veterinary surgeons are one of the first points of call for advice regarding a dog's behaviour. If an owner's concern or the way a dog behaves in the surgery in any way runs the risk of contributing to a dog bite incident, it is incumbent upon attending staff to intervene by ensuring the clients are given expert preventative advice. This should *not* entail implying that a dog displaying fear and anxiety-based aggression in the surgery is a dangerous dog and should be treated as such, as has been the attitude among certain veterinary quarters in the past. Rather than jumping immediately to alarmist conclusions, there should be sympathetic and non-judgemental discussion about any other contexts outside the veterinary realm in which fear or aggression may be displayed. If authoritative advice is not available in-house, clients should be offered referral elsewhere. Cost should not be made an obstacle to being given essential advice – hence the ideal situation where all veterinary staff are cognisant of accurate behavioural basics.

Aggressive responses created by veterinary attention itself are sins of commission. Failing to ensure correct advice is given when needed and in a timely manner should be considered a sin of omission. (Shepherd 2020)

As we can see from the ramifications of UK 'dangerous dogs' legislation, **euthanasia** of dogs is often required (both justified and completely unnecessary) and must be carried out by a veterinary surgeon. Such euthanasia may be ordered by the court in which case a court order to this effect will be available and should be provided by those requesting that it is carried out (generally a police officer). It is however the case that euthanasia has been carried out in certain situations which has subsequently been deemed to have been unlawful.

Although there is no legal requirement for owners of such dogs to be informed that their dog has been put to sleep, the moral and ethical veterinary obligation should extend further than the law requires. There are not infrequent cases where euthanasia is carried out without the knowledge or consent of the owner in addition to being unlawful. Delays in the court appeal process, mislaid paperwork and mistakes made regarding their identity result in dogs being 'accidentally' killed. I have recently arrived at kennels where two companion dogs were housed, with the plan that one of the dogs should be involved in the behaviour assessment of the other. To my dismay and the owners' grief and outrage, one of the dogs was already dead. The buck stops with the veterinary surgeon wielding the syringe whose responsibility it must be to avoid such tragic errors.

Apart from the dogs which their owners have 'signed over' (the police becoming the effective owners) *all* dogs seized and kept in custody have owners who should be accorded the same respect regarding their pet as any other client. If veterinary surgeons are themselves not to fall foul of the law, it is essential that they do all in their power to ensure that their imminent irreversible action is lawful and that the owners of the dogs have been made fully aware of it.

For further information regarding unlawful euthanasia please follow the link https://parrywelchlacey.wordpress.com/2020/06/11/euthanasia-of-dogs-without-consent/.

VETS AND THE ANIMAL WELFARE ACT

Prior to the passing of the Animal Welfare Act in 2006, animal welfare law was largely reactive. Action could only be taken once an animal had suffered unnecessarily. The Animal Welfare Act 2006 by contrast stipulates that there is an obligation not only not to cause suffering but to prevent it. It encompasses both physical and mental suffering and states that this obligation extends beyond the owner of the animal to anyone who may be considered to have a responsibility towards it. In earlier incarnations of the legislation, it had to be shown that suffering had already occurred before a case could be made out, whereas we now have to be more predictive and proactive regarding conditions which are likely to cause an animal to suffer. It also divides suffering into 'necessary' and 'unnecessary', acknowledging that certain procedures and conditions to which animals are routinely subjected entail a degree of suffering.

In a letter to the *Veterinary Record* in 2015, Dr. John Bradshaw, Director of the Bristol Anthrozoology Institute, highlighted the responsibility that veterinary surgeons ought to have to prevent mental suffering in animals and questioned why, at that time, less than 0.1% of UK practising veterinary surgeons specialised in behaviour (VR, Dec 5th 2015). In the same issue, Professor Daniel Mills, as quoted from his lecture at the BVA Congress that year, considered that dogs 'work hard to fit in and please their owners' but questioned whether we as humans 'keep our side of the bargain'. Peter Sandoe of Copenhagen University further suggested in his presentation that '(human) love does not automatically equate to good welfare for a pet animal'.

In my reply (VR Dec 19th 2015) while I wholeheartedly agreed with Dr Bradshaw's concern regarding the lack of veterinary interest in behaviour as a specialism, I considered that routine consideration of behavioural health within general veterinary practice was, in my view, equally important. A dog's welfare should encompass both physical and mental state and, as such, behaviour and welfare were inextricably linked.

I went on to question whether there was fundamental difference between the profession's perception of, and obligation towards, firstly, dogs that were distressed by thunderstorms or by separation from their owner and, secondly, dogs that were distressed by veterinary handling. Both could be considered examples of poor mental welfare: the first, an anxious and fearful dog in need of behavioural assistance and yet the second, a 'dangerous' creature whose owners, at the very least, should be made aware of the legal risks. Other correspondence in the *Veterinary Times* had voiced the extreme polarisation of views on the subject (Darryl Thorpe 'Zero-tolerance policy on aggressive dogs' VT Sept 7th 2015 and Carol McGuigan 'We shouldn't wash our hands of aggressive dogs' VT Oct 5th 2015).

Clearly, a middle road needed to be found whereby veterinary surgeons could keep themselves and their staff safe as well as abide by their professional obligations to the RCVS code of conduct and legal obligations under the Animal Welfare Act, in providing equal care for the mental, as well as physical, health of their patients.

When owners seek veterinary advice, apart from in cases of obvious injury, they are concerned about the animal because their **behaviour** has in some way changed. Behavioural symptoms are taken as indicators of physiological abnormality and disease. Although fearfulness and aggression are obvious behavioural symptoms, physical signs such as lethargy, limping, coughing and vomiting also involve changes in behaviour, the presence of which may indicate physical malaise. All veterinary examination and diagnosis must therefore involve assessing behavioural change and its implications for underlying disease. If such examination indicates the need for veterinary intervention, then it is our obligation to provide it by offering advice and, if necessary, further investigation and medical or surgical intervention. **The same obligation exists for potential welfare cases and concerns and there is a need for an animal's behaviour to be considered throughout.**

But what is suffering? According to a paper published in the *Veterinary Record* (Baumgaertner et al. 2016) which reviewed veterinary expert reports prepared for court purposes, the reports typically contained much inconsistency and ambiguity regarding what suffering actually was. Observations highlighted included the following:

- the lack of, or variable, definitions of suffering
- variable or absent reference to mental as well as physical suffering
- the assumption of suffering owing to the presence of medical conditions
- a degree of anthropomorphism
- dispute regarding the relationship between physical findings and suffering
- general poor use of up-to-date references

David Morton's editorial comment in the same issue (VR Sept 2016) provided some assistance by stating, 'Physical suffering may be inferred from external examinations, post mortem findings, laboratory reports, and other parameters of health and well-being. Mental suffering is different and relies more on an assessment of the behaviour of an animal reflecting its internal emotions and adverse feelings at a point in time.' He stated further that, in his view, '*the behaviour of an animal provides one of the gold standards of a welfare assessment, despite its inherent difficulties*' (emphasis added). James Yeates (VR Feb 2017) commented that the various definitions of suffering may be practically simplified to 'experience, or be subjected to something bad or unpleasant'.

It is therefore quite clear that even if the preceding chapters have not proved persuasive, to fulfil one's legal (as well as professional) obligations, a modicum of knowledge regarding what dogs do and why they do it is essential. Insight is required into how emotions, both positive and negative, are reflected in the behaviour of dogs. In turn, the behaviour of dogs provides the means by which their welfare and quality of life can be assessed.

12 Legal cases to demonstrate behavioural principles

A SALUTARY TALE

At the age of 5½, my son was bitten by a dog. We were at the house of acquaintances, who had sold up to move abroad and were having an 'open-house' farewell party. They were in their early sixties with two adult daughters and the dog in question was 14 years old, partially sighted and deaf. He had been in the garden begging at my older daughter's feet for a share of her plate when my son approached and patted him on the head. As far as my son was concerned, a friendly overture; to the dog, an unjustified challenge – 'my food and you're not having it'.

Our hosts were shocked. The often-repeated phrase 'He's never done that before' was both bandied about and believed as well as the warning-bell excuse that the dog was never usually approached while eating. Had this therefore been a mundane occurrence – grist to the mill of any behaviour counsellor? Or a life-altering trauma for all concerned – a death knoll for a dog with a previously unblotted copybook? Was the dog 'dangerous' or had he, in reality, never been 'safe' but simply, in his life experience, insufficiently tested?

The consequences were, by luck rather than good judgement, relatively mild. Although wheals were evident from eyebrow to lip and with a small puncture inside the mouth, my son's cries, ostensibly of pain but mainly of indignant incomprehension that a dog could behave thus, were soon soothed with offered sweets and toys. On the premise that one should get back on a horse immediately after falling off, I insisted that he ask the dog to sit and give it a titbit and tried to counter his protestations that the dog was 'stupid'.

After all, for my son, the episode had been a learning experience on a par with being burnt by an illicitly struck match or falling off the back of a chair, having being told for the umpteenth time to sit still. Or was it? Do we muzzle or destroy matches and chairs? Are the owners of such offending articles dragged before the courts? What makes the dog an exception?

The rare occasion when one, as a veterinary surgeon, sees animal-related occurrences, even momentarily, from the perspective of the general public is always a salutary experience. How should one react? What is 'the norm'? Although I found myself instantly analysing the situation as a vet and behaviour counsellor, my emotions as a mother interfered with rational thought. The questions rushed to be answered. What had my son done to provoke the attack? Would he be scarred? Did my friends know their dog could behave like this? Should I have seen it coming? Had I misled my son into thinking that all dogs could be foil to an imaginary light

149

sabre as ours were at home? My reactions could have varied from instant demands for euthanasia, to reporting the dog to the police as 'dangerous' or to immediate punitive retaliation towards the dog so that he should learn 'not to do it again'.

As it was, politeness and the British stiff upper lip prevailed, and the bite remained an unreported statistic. My son returned home with the same cavalier attitude to his own dogs as he had had previously, but with a slightly healthier respect for those he didn't know. His partner in mishap retired to France to be kept out of the vicinity of small children and food. (Written in 2004)

INTRODUCTION

The legal cases discussed here all highlight some aspect of the misunderstanding of dogs and inadequacies of the law in preventing injury by dogs, primarily by biting. I have been personally involved as an expert witness in all of them. They illustrate topics such as the true meaning of obedience, the erroneous belief in dominance, the lack of awareness of human conflict on a dog's emotions and the nature of reward and punishment from the canine point of view. Together with simple lack of foresight, these misunderstandings have all contributed to dog owners falling foul of the law. The cases are intended to underpin the information and ideas I have presented thus far and to emphasise yet again how early and knowledgeable veterinary intervention regarding the behaviour of dogs can raise awareness and help to prevent future mishap. Two cases also highlight the link between pain and aggression and how early veterinary diagnosis and treatment are essential.

They are also evidence of how and why current reliance on human prosecution and punishment without education is doomed to failure. Reality of life and the welfare implications for dogs while confined in police-contracted kennels 'to ensure public safety' are also revealed. The urgent need for re-education regarding dogs is not confined solely to the dog-owning public but all those occupied in dog-related employment. Without this, there is the very real risk that the behaviour of dogs seized under the Dangerous Dogs Act deteriorates to the extent that labelling a dog as 'dangerous' becomes a self-fulfilling prophecy.

I have used my own dogs in assessments; a Jack Russell terrier and two lurchers, all neutered females.[1]

The cases involve the following:

1. Overdependence on physical control
2. Misunderstanding of obedience
3. Significance of veterinary history – two cases
4. Bad human behaviour
5. Redirected aggression
6. Misdirected play
7. Conflict with police

---

[1] Whenever 'my assistant' is mentioned, this refers to my long-standing and long-suffering partner Rod, who has provided much needed practical and emotional support for many years.

1.   OVER-DEPENDENCE ON PHYSICAL CONTROL

A 3½-year-old entire male German Shepherd dog called Donnie, while being used as a security patrol dog, had become briefly out of his male owner's control while on duty and had chased and allegedly bitten the leg of a teenager. His owner was duly charged with an offence under Section 3 of the Dangerous Dogs Act. The dog was allowed to remain at home while awaiting court proceedings.

Donnie was described as a friendly pet dog at home, good with resident and visiting young children, thoroughly house trained and seldom disobedient. He was frightened of fireworks, when he hid under the kitchen table, and often tried to chase bicycles. **He had never been allowed off lead as his owner had had no training at all in off-lead control and was 'not sure of what Donnie would do'.**

Donnie's history was as follows, much of which was gleaned during a home visit to assess the dog *in situ*. He had been purchased from a police dog handler a year previously to be used as a 'deterrent' dog for his owner's future role as a security patrol guard. His owner, a novice dog handler, subsequently underwent National Association of Security Dog Users (NASDU) training for on-lead patrol and deterrent work only. This training relied solely on the contrast between jerked lead, applied choke chain and verbal correction as punishments and a game with a toy as a reward. An additional requirement of the borough council where he worked was that the dog should be muzzled while on patrol. Unfortunately, his owner was instructed by a fellow trainer to use a tight fabric muzzle, which prevented Donnie panting as well as barking effectively. He was described, unsurprisingly, as 'not enjoying' having the muzzle put on. In addition, as I was forced to point out early in the assessment, he could not possibly predict the positive reward of play while wearing a muzzle. Donnie's obedience while working was therefore entirely based on the presence or absence of physical punishment.

When on duty, he barked as best he could in a defensive manner when feeling threatened and might pull towards the source of the threat, the 'deterrent' aspect of his duties. Donnie became excited when visitors arrived at the home but had never shown aggression or threat in an 'off-duty' context.

When visiting to assess Donnie, I ascertained the exact details of the offence. These were that, upon opening the transport cage door, Donnie had leapt out of the cage before his handler could put him on lead or secure his muzzle. He immediately chased, and allegedly bit, one of two approaching rather rowdy teenagers. He stopped immediately when his owner shouted at him.

He was extremely obedient and tolerant throughout the assessment in normal off-duty contexts. However, remembering that Donnie's protection training did not extend to off-lead chase and grab/restraint, I asked his owner to behave exactly as he and Donnie had been trained to do if approached by a potential assailant. Donnie was first fitted with a muzzle and kept on choke chain and lead as was required. As long as I, acting as a potential assailant, obeyed instruction to not come any closer, Donnie remained sitting at his owner's feet. If I ignored this and continued to approach in a threatening manner, Donnie sprang at my right arm several times and would have grabbed it if the muzzle had not been in place. In so doing, however, he showed no animosity and I could personally remove the muzzle immediately afterwards to engage him in friendly social interaction.

OBSERVATIONS AND CONCLUSIONS

Donnie had been trained on lead almost entirely using punishment/negative re-inforcement contrast. This was supplied by the application and contrasting release of the choke chain. Although a game with a toy was used in training sessions as a rewarding event, such a reward could not be used at all when he was muzzled and on duty. While in training, such a dog may well maintain a more positive emotional state and grab a stooge's arm in much the same way as it would a thrown ball. When working, however, Donnie was subjected to unpredictable threats on a routine basis and had received no positive reward to help counteract emotional deterioration. There was a risk that such a dog would react aggressively out of worsening fear and uncertainty.

In common with a number of protection or attack dogs, Donnie, I believed, was extremely confused regarding human requirements of him. He had been encouraged to bark and lunge at certain people in order to appear intimidating. At the very same time, in order for his handler to maintain control of him, he will have been punished via the lead and choke chain for doing exactly these behaviours. In addition, the unpleasant sensation deliberately produced by the choke chain will have made negative associations with any context in which the chain was used.

His owner, through no fault of his own, had been given insufficient instruction (if any) in controlling his dog off lead. From a behavioural perspective, off-lead control should always be established *before* transferring command information to a restraining lead. Relying solely on a lead for control inevitably means that the guidance any dog needs will be completely absent if a dog suddenly finds him-self free.

He also had the false belief that Donnie would act in defence only upon his verbal command. In reality, the information upon which any dog bases his decisions includes the whole environmental context in which the command is given. My assessment confirmed that the threatening approach of a person who disobeyed his handler's instructions to keep at a distance was the salient feature to which Donnie responded rather than a verbal command. In any dog trained to view certain people as threatening and respond accordingly, an effective and reliable 'don't attack yet' command is as, if not more, important than an 'attack now' command.

Donnie's behaviour during the incident was the result of a combination of un-foreseen circumstances, namely,

- Alarm at the approaching noise and what it might signify to him
- Chase behaviour stimulated by noise, waving arms and running of the alleged victim
- Owing to momentary lack of physical control by his handler, suddenly finding himself free without his accustomed restraint, muzzle or command to im-mediately do as his emotions dictated

It was unlikely that Donnie, as he ran forward, intended to bite, merely to appear threatening as he had been trained to do. During the assessment, when deliberately put into a situation for which he had been trained and prepared, he made specific attempts to take hold of my right arm only. Although it may have been more likely that he would make similar moves if acting without command, it was not possible to say categorically that another part of a person's anatomy would not be accidentally targeted.

I commented that it was surprising to me and a credit to Donnie's good nature that, despite such conflicting training, Donnie remained an extremely well-disposed dog towards people and one who would much prefer, in any social situation, to play rather than attack.

Finally, I did not consider Donnie to be a dangerous dog nor one who would, entirely without provocation, have any intention of injuring a human being. He had, however, been trained to assume that, against his better nature, grabbing and holding onto parts of the human body was at times the required thing to do.

By the conclusion of the court case, his owner was considering keeping Donnie as a pet dog and finding alternative employment.

2.   MISUNDERSTANDING OF OBEDIENCE

A female dog owner was charged in 2017 under the Animal Welfare Act 2006. She had been seen punching and kicking her mixed breed dog while in a drunken state and was subsequently arrested and charged with animal abuse. Her dog, Sasha, was taken into custody. Unusually, I was instructed to carry out an assessment of the owner while in the presence of her dog and their interaction.

I duly obtained all relevant documentation, including a completed questionnaire regarding Sasha from her owner. Sasha had been owned since puppyhood and had not had any conventional dog training. She was, however, reported to be house trained, non-destructive, friendly towards people and other dogs and generally 'behaving well' on or off lead. She was however also described as being 'stubborn' at times (with all the connotations this word embodies as previously described in Chapter 5).

THE ASSESSMENT

Possibly contrary to expectations of the charging authorities, it was immediately obvious how delighted dog and owner were to see each other after six months of separation. There was no hint of wariness on the part of the dog, simply extremely enthusiastic recognition and greeting.

Very early on during the assessment, it became clear that her owner became frustrated with Sasha if she did not obey her and she proceeded to use physical prompts such as pushing her rump down to sit and raising her voice if she did not comply. I commented in my report that this was an almost universal human response if owners had not been shown how to guide a dog's choices without the need for threat or coercion.

Questioning the owner revealed that it was Sasha's 'disobedience' in not coming to her when called which had made her most frustrated and angry and that she was in the habit of using physical reprimand and coercion to 'make Sasha move' when she didn't want to.

I showed her how the dual use food and reduction of threat was immediately successful in getting Sasha to come to her and sit immediately on command. I explained that, if threatened, an instinctive behaviour in any dog's repertoire was to stay still or move away. If commands entailed threat, particularly on the recall, the strategy to stay away was the obvious choice from Sasha's point of view rather than the obedience that the owner required. Stubborn simply meant that a dog at that moment was not doing what an owner wanted her to do. It was one of the most common complaints made among dog owners.

I encouraged her throughout the assessment to discontinue using a pointing gesture or any body movements that implied threat to Sasha. Her owner could immediately understand how her previous means of communication had been at best confusing, and at worst threatening, to her dog.

CONCLUSIONS

I believed that my explanation and demonstration had been a light bulb moment for Sasha's owner, as for the vast majority of other dog owners who were frustrated by their dog's lack of obedience. Indeed, it was still all too common for owners to believe that 'dominance' and coercion were all that dogs understood in order to obey and that punishment for disobedience was essential.

I observed that, when inebriated, habitual human behaviour tended to get worse. I believed that, drunk as the owner accepted she was at the time of the incident, her behaviour was an extreme version of how she believed dogs had to be dealt with, namely, coerced into obedience and punished for disobedience.

I understood that she had now fully complied with an alcohol rehabilitation programme and had not drunk alcohol for many months.

In my view, she was genuinely remorseful for the way she had misunderstood dogs in general, and consequently treated Sasha specifically, in the past. I also believed that her declared aim of having Sasha returned to her was a primary motive for abstinence from alcohol. Denying the return of the dog might have the opposite effect.

Sasha was allowed to be returned to her tearful owner, who up to the time of writing, continues to remain completely sober.

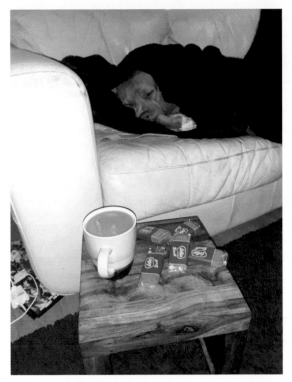

Sasha in May 2020 during corona virus outbreak.

3.   THE SIGNIFICANCE OF VET HISTORY

A   6-YEAR-OLD MALE NEUTERED ROTTWEILER CALLED TYSON

Tyson was rehomed at the age of 14 months as a neglected dog. He lived with an adult male owner, the owner's brother and their parents. The father had suffered a stroke two years previously and had regular carer visits. An assessment was required because in July 2015 Tyson had been involved in a scuffle with two other dogs and a month later in August 2015 he had bitten a visiting carer on her arm. The assessment did not take place until the end of August 2016, a year later. Before both these incidents, Tyson was already under a Court Order from 2013 to be kept muzzled (a fabric type was used habitually on walks) and on lead in public following an 'attack' on a Dachshund.

Tyson had not been taken to training classes but was considered to be clever and well trained at home. He was known to be wary and nervous of strangers and to want to investigate other dogs. His owner had complied with the 2013 court order apart from the one incidence of accidental escape in July 2015 as he was being prepared to go for a walk. Further information gleaned from the witness statements and during the assessment included that the bite to the carer occurred while in the back garden. The owner asserted that she had been told not to touch Tyson but a dispute had arisen as to whether Tyson had simply bitten 'out of the blue' after sniffing her or after she put her arms over his head and round his neck.

As ever, the purpose of the assessment was the following:

- provide a rationale for the alleged incident
- give an opinion as to whether the dog was a danger to public safety
- determine what precautions needed to be put in place to achieve this

To investigate thoroughly and provide both mitigation for his actions and a prognosis (although not strictly considered necessary for court purposes), it was essential to take Tyson's informative veterinary history into account, obtained after the assessment.

SUMMARY OF VETERINARY HISTORY OBTAINED

In June 2014, a house call was requested as Tyson was having difficulty standing up. He had to be muzzled for examination when he growled specifically on extension of his hips. Comment was made that he 'might need x-ray of hips and stifles'.

He received a booster vaccination 9th June 2015 and was muzzled for examination.

On 29th March 2016, the veterinary records first mentioned the previous control order from 2013 and also the impending court cases regarding the incidents in July and August 2015.

On 11th August 2016, Tyson needed a booster vaccination but a 'hot spot' on his head was reported. Owner then questioned whether 'injections could make him aggressive as by now he was growling at any stranger in the house if (they) stroked him on the head'.

The 'hot spot' was later clipped under sedation and corticosteroids were prescribed.

There was a mention on 29th Sept 2016 (following the assessment and receipt of my report) that 'Kendal Shepherd mentioned to owner that hips and stifles should be x-rayed as aggression may be due to discomfort'.

COMMENTS ON ROTTWEILER BREED

Historically, the breed came into existence as a droving dog, and as such was expected to be very tolerant of strangers in general but to react in a protective and potentially sudden manner (with no warning preamble) should they come into close proximity of the dog or perceived possessions. Such dogs are able to lull people into a false sense of security. The breed description as 'good natured, not nervous or aggressive' is at odds with the acceptance of 'natural guarding instincts'. Dogs only have warning signals such as growling or threatened aggression with which to express their natural guarding instincts. Owners cannot be blamed for any misperception of this complimentary but behaviourally ambivalent description.

COMMENTS ON THE ASSESSMENT TAKEN FROM MY REPORT

Tyson was exceptionally obedient to both his owner and his mother both in and out of the house and in the face of distractions such as traffic, cyclists, passers-by and other dogs.

He was a very vocal dog, growling habitually as befits his breed. His family were used to his vocalisations when playing and did not view them necessarily as a sign of warning or impending aggression. However, as shown during the assessment, he could also growl as a warning when he felt under threat.

I wrote in the report:

Tyson is a dog who does not tolerate intimate handling from a stranger, most specifically in a veterinary context. This is a not uncommon finding in dogs which historically have associated stranger handling with pain and discomfort. When held and restrained during the assessment, his defensive growling was more pronounced.

Over the last four years, Tyson has become progressively wary and potentially aggressive at the veterinary surgery. Unfortunately, owing to lack of awareness of the negative effects of veterinary handling, often associated with discomfort, this finding is all too common. He has suffered with vaccine reactions in the past as well as lameness which have necessitated close veterinary attention and restraint, accompanied by injections. He has growled on restraint and limb manipulation during a house call two years ago when he appeared to have difficulty standing up and was in pain. He can yelp if patted on the rump.

(In hindsight, one has to question the wisdom of administering steroids with their now well-known side effects, including aggression, to such a dog. Notari and Mills 2015)

It is unfortunately my experience that in the absence of expert advice, courts do not specify the kind of muzzle that should be worn to be both secure and humane in the event of a muzzling control order. A fabric muzzle if tight enough to prevent a bite, is inhumane in that a dog cannot pant or drink. His owner cannot be blamed for this. The basket type muzzle as now used ought to be recommended consistently.

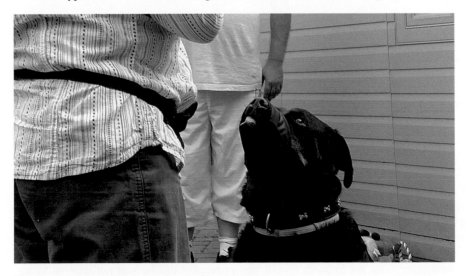

Tyson wearing fabric muzzle, unable to pant.

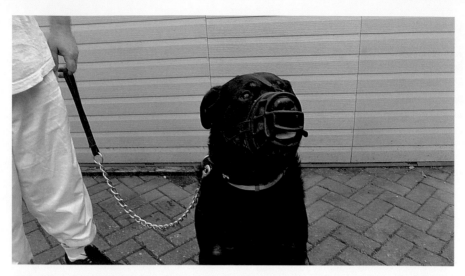

Tyson wearing basket muzzle and able to pant.

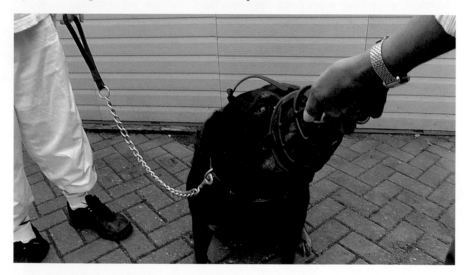

Tyson being given food through basket muzzle.

CONCLUSIONS

I found no evidence that Tyson would bite unless physical contact and restraint were imposed on him. I was therefore more persuaded by the owner's version of events, that the carer was likely to have tried to hug him, in spite of being told not to touch him, rather than the bite coming out of the blue.

Recommendations were that Tyson was to be kept away from visitors unable to follow instructions not to touch him. It was imperative that he was not allowed to accidentally escape from house again. I was of the opinion that, under the existing control measures and with a suitable muzzle, Tyson did not present a danger to public safety.

POST-SCRIPT

Further veterinary history for Tyson has recently been obtained. Around the time of the case coming to court (April 2017), radiography of his hips and stifles were again discussed but comment is made that, as by that time the bite incident had occurred nearly two years previously, 'it would be difficult to say whether (the dog had been in) discomfort then'. By November 2017, Tyson still growled profusely on 'limited' examination but the possibility of medication was mentioned only 'if hind limb gait worsens'. By December 2019, a dietary joint supplement was being given but had not helped a developing foreleg lameness. For the first time, non-steroidal anti-inflammatory medication was prescribed. There is no record of any radiographic investigation or diagnosis ever being carried out.

Much as it pains me to criticise veterinary colleagues, there are glaring omissions in Tyson's history, when looked at as a whole. He was unable to stand and in pain in 2014 when growling on examination was first mentioned. X-rays of hips and stifles were recommended then but not followed up, neither was my own recommendation in 2016. Despite the assumption in 2017 that a cause of pain could not be diagnosed in retrospect, one could surely hazard a guess, with this history, that pain had been present throughout. It appears that the physical symptom of lameness was the only criterion by which Tyson's discomfort was measured and aggression as a behavioural symptom discounted. This case highlights the necessity to consider pain even in the absence of lameness and investigate properly all dogs who become aggressive for the first time on examination of specific joints. This is even more important in breeds predisposed to orthopaedic conditions.

B Male long-haired German Shepherd called Beau

I assessed Beau twice – once when he was 17 months old and again at the age of 5 years. He had been taken into in the custody of the police on both occasions. His story illustrates several failures. The over-arching failure was of the legislation in preventing offending, in dogs in general and in the case of Beau specifically. When analysed, individual failures, almost all 'crimes of omission', could be identified on the part of:

a.   the owner and her family.
b.   those who 'cared' for him in police-contracted kennels.
c.   Beau's attending veterinary surgeons.

Beau was living with his adult female owner at the time of the first offence but had moved to live with her parents thereafter, when her father was mainly responsible for his exercise.

The dog first came to the attention of the police when, at home alone, Beau escaped through a patio door which appeared to have been left ajar and was alleged to have bitten a next-door neighbour. At that time, the history I was given was that he had been purchased from a reputable GSD (German Shepherd Dog) breeder, was registered with a veterinary surgery and was microchipped and insured. He had attended puppy classes, had one-to-one training at home and was considered to be a obedient, house trained and non-destructive dog. His recall was reliable and he could be safely let off lead in the presence of other people and dogs. At this point, no aggression had been seen, but he was described as being 'protective' of his owner in that he barked at certain people when out for a walk with her. He was recognised as being initially wary of strangers but 'making friends' readily. He was 'sensitive' to handling round his back legs.

Veterinary history was not sought on this occasion, but on reviewing it later following the second incident, it was noted on his records in June 2013 (when 6 months old) that he was presented for general malaise and found hard to examine as 'so playful'. During the examination, he progressed to 'play biting' and was muzzled eventually as he was 'curling his lip' and snapping.

Upon seizure by police officers, he was said to have become 'aggressive', though what form this took was never specified, and had required pepper spray and a dog catch pole to restrain him.

Unusually, I was allowed into the holding kennels to assess Beau in August 2014.

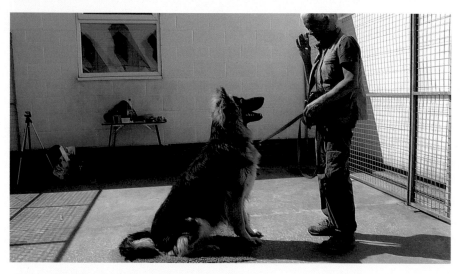

Beau demonstrating his obedience to 'sit', 'down' and 'watch me'.

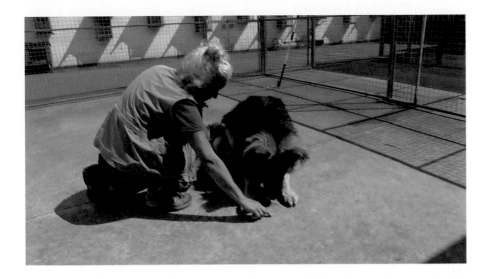

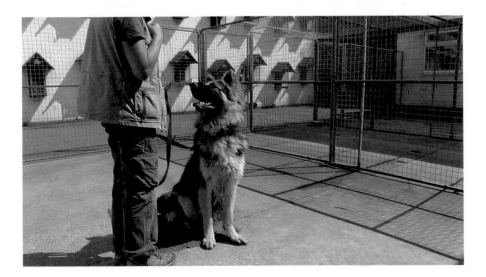

The observations and recommendations after my first assessment were the following:

In his general demeanour and behaviour, Beau is very much typical of his breed. He is observant, reactive, vocal, highly trainable and initially wary of strangers, particularly men. Indeed, it is these typical breed-specific traits which dictate that the German shepherd dog is the working dog of choice for the police force and military. As they are innately wary, it is relatively easy to utilise this negative emotion to train a 'protective' dog. Such training happens deliberately in a working dog, but frequently accidentally in the pet dog. Barking at passers-by is inadvertently rewarded by the apparently obedient departure of the passer-by and the cessation of perceived threat. It therefore accidently becomes the behaviour of choice. Should a passer-by not pass by but approach instead, a postman for example, then the threat to the dog increases with a potential increase in the perceived need for defence.

During the assessment, Beau showed no hint of aggression unless he himself felt threatened in some way. His distinct preference even when threatened is to retreat to avoid engagement, as he did when I entered his kennel. If however he is unable to retreat, for example when restrained on lead or behind bars, then his behaviour will become more overtly aggressive. He showed very mild defensive aggression during the veterinary examination and, when Rod paid him direct attention, in particular when he reached a hand towards him, expressed his wariness by barking. He did not show any overt aggression towards him but could be encouraged, by Rod deliberately threatening him, to become more vigorous in his defence.

He is, however, a very forgiving dog whose emotions and perception of danger are easily changed if the behaviour of those around him changes. He is therefore quickly able to learn good things about people, supporting his owner's view that, once introduced to strangers in a pleasant way, he quickly becomes tolerant and friendly towards them. However, the opposite side of this behavioural coin is that he can equally quickly learn that barking and threatening behaviour is the most efficient way of ridding him of threat, hence the ease with which his breed can be trained to bark at, chase and grab people.

I am concerned that, unless the kennel staff make concerted efforts to present themselves in a non-threatening and informative way to Beau, this damaging learning process will continue in confinement, where Beau is feeling more or less continually under threat. (emphasis original)

History shows that this concern was more than justified.

RECOMMENDATIONS

I had been informed that Beau's owner was now living with her parents, who had another dog and whose property was thoroughly secure, and that this was where Beau would live once released. I urged the court and the police to consider allowing Beau home to live with her and her parents under an interim Control Order until such a time as the matter was finally resolved. I did not believe that Beau presented a danger to the public given informed guidance and supervision. Furthermore, I believed (at the time) the owner and her family to be thoroughly responsible, who were capable of giving such guidance and supervision and who would follow any restrictions imposed to the letter.

It was essential that Beau was not given the opportunity to be outside his premises unaccompanied in the future, with no-one present to guide his behaviour. I did not feel that a muzzling order was required as there was no evidence that, when in the presence of his owner or her father, Beau had ever behaved inappropriately in the past. I pointed out that, in any event, dogs did not put on their own muzzles before escaping from their home, so the prevention of such escape was of the essence.

I emphasised that, on his release, Beau might need some remedial training to counter his memories of kennels even after this relatively short confinement, compared unfortunately to many seized dogs. I would be happy to give further advice to his owner if needed but it appeared she was already in the hands of Beau's previous trainer.

On his return from police kennels in September 2014, he was taken for veterinary examination a day later as was found to be lame on his right foreleg. He was described variously as 'nervous', 'excited and jumpy', 'barking and showing teeth' and 'agitated' and was again muzzled.

He was booked in for castration two weeks later, but which did not take place until April 2017.

By the time of the second incident in November 2017, Beau was living with the owner's parents, while she visited regularly to assist in exercising him. There he lived with a companion dog and, as a headcollar had been advised for this dog, Beau routinely wore one also. In brief, both dogs were being walked together in the evening by the owner and her father. While faeces from the companion dog were being cleared up, the adult female victim approached from behind, startling his owner and Beau who sprang forward and bit her left torso.

He was by this time described as 'very nervous, anxious and reactive' and who routinely barked at several features of the environment – male strangers who entered the house, birds, squirrels, the next-door neighbours and the window cleaner. He became very insecure if even momentarily separated from those he was bonded to, particularly his female owner. He also reacted to loud noises, such as fireworks, and had in the past barked at the Hoover, although this particular aspect of his behaviour was said to have been successfully addressed by the owner's mother.

According to his veterinary records, Beau had become progressively even harder to handle, being by then perceived as a thoroughly aggressive dog who could not be handled at all for full examination, even when muzzled. There was no evidence whatsoever throughout his veterinary history that any attempt had been made in-house to address this issue and the impact on his mental welfare, let alone any acknowledgement of the 'knock-on effect' into the public arena. It was also noted that, at home, Beau was difficult to groom all over, particularly his hind legs, but the owner's father was more successful than she was. Again, this issue had not been addressed.

Apart from training received earlier at puppy and agility classes as well as on a one-to-one basis, Beau had also received training from the owner of the kennels at which he occasionally boarded. I was made aware from the pre-assessment behaviour questionnaire that there were disagreements between the owner's parents as to how best to correct Beau's behaviour. It appeared that these arose from certain inconsistencies in opinion as to what Beau should be allowed to do, such as go upstairs, get on the furniture or be given treats if agitated by fireworks.

THE SECOND ASSESSMENT

On attending police kennels for the second time to assess Beau in November 2018 (11 months after the incident), I was informed by his kennel records, which I was allowed to see, that Beau had only been taken out of his kennel for exercise and for veterinary attention on a rigid dog pole, owing to the risk he was thought to pose. He had been muzzled for veterinary treatment, such as vaccination, and for unsuccessful attempts to groom him and remove matted parts of his fur, owing to his intolerance of close handling.

Contrary to what one might be led to believe from the kennel records, it took me a matter of minutes to lead Beau out of his kennel restrained only on a slip lead. The assessment was video-recorded as routine and the following is a description of how this was achieved.

"I was first led to the sleeping quarters of his kennel. The metal sheet on the door to the sleeping quarters precluded full visibility, both for me and Beau. He was barking vigorously, as were many other dogs. I felt it safer, and to give Beau more space, that he should be confined in the larger 'run' end of the kennel for me to communicate with him. We therefore moved round to the run side of the kennel block, while a member of kennel staff remained poised to shut the guillotine door between the kennel sections, as soon as Beau entered the run.

Still barking vigorously, although not just at me, Beau was unwilling to venture out of his sleeping quarters towards me. After a short while, he began to take food titbits thrown towards him as he became a little bolder. At this point, he was showing a classic **'approach-avoidance' emotional conflict**, in that he wanted the food but did not want to approach me to get it. As I did not feel under threat from him and could recognise his underlying fear, I tested his response by opening the kennel door and to begin with, standing, then crouching, in the entrance. Beau would not respond to his name nor approach me. As he showed no intent to rush towards me, I deemed it safe to enter the kennel fully, with the door held shut behind me by Rod. Very soon, Beau began to come a little further out from the sleeping quarters, in order to reach thrown food titbits, but then retreated again to bark from inside.

About 5 minutes 10 seconds after my first approach, I asked the attending police officer and Rod to move away out of Beau's direct sight lines as I felt their presence may be hindering progress. Almost immediately Beau stopped barking, stood with gently wagging tail and then came out of the sleeping end to reach the food titbits just long enough for the guillotine door to be dropped shut behind him.

I immediately began to engage Beau in simple obedience tasks (emotional stabilisers), such as to sit and to give each paw to shake in turn. He was compliant, showed no aggression towards me and took food gently from the hand. At 6 minutes 16 seconds, I placed a slip lead over his head. He pulled away slightly from this restraint, but it was easy to re-engage him in a request to sit. I then led him out of the kennel and into the secure enclosure for the rest of the assessment. I advised Rod to stay outside and film from there until I had had a little more time with Beau on my own.

After my assessment I commented:

Throughout the assessment, Beau showed no aggression towards me but was reactive to certain events, such as being scanned for a microchip. As described by his owner, he has become fearful and potentially aggressive to male strangers visiting the house.

This was confirmed by my assessment in his responses to my male assistant. He is extremely alert to any changes in his environment yet despite this, he remains a highly trainable and responsive dog.

It is highly likely that all his 'less than desirable' behaviours will have been rehearsed in kennels since his seizure in January 2018. Despite the assumption that he cannot be handled without restraint on a rigid dog pole, my assessment shows otherwise. I am aware of the effect on people that anticipation of a dog's 'aggressive' or untoward behaviour of any kind tends to become a self-fulfilling prophecy. **With the greatest respect for kennel staff, the perceived need for pole restraint, muzzling and the need to 'wrestle with a lion', as stated in the kennel records, is at great risk of creating the very response in Beau that one wants to avoid.**

Regarding Beau's owner and current management system, I am concerned over certain matters, taking into account the amount of training and behaviour advice received by his owner since a puppy. I have had details of certain inconsistencies in the approach to Beau's training and control. I would like to be assured, from now on, that these have been resolved and that there are no other contexts in which Beau may be receiving mixed messages, which may be hindering progress. **His behaviour at the veterinary surgery has deteriorated over time although the reasons for this cannot be laid solely at his owner's door. I wonder whether this issue has been specifically addressed for future welfare and veterinary care, and also why his owner is still not able to fully groom him all over.**

If past advice has been sound, then one must question whether it has been followed to the letter in a consistent manner, by all those in charge of Beau. If advice given thus far has, on the other hand, been ill-advised or has not covered all aspects of his behaviour, then I would be happy to give further behaviour and training advice.

Beau is a very affectionate yet extremely emotionally insecure dog much in need of constant human guidance. He cannot be expected to make appropriate decisions for himself, as much as we expect, and take for granted, most dogs to do. In the absence of consistent pre-emptive guidance, I believe that Beau now needs to be muzzled in public, preferably in combination with secure head control. This alone cannot be relied upon to prevent misdemeanour and must be accompanied by confident, meaningful and educational handler guidance. I have just become aware of a custom-made device, which incorporates both muzzle and head harness and has very recently become available, which I believe would be very suitable for Beau should the court see fit to allow him to return to his owner.

A subsequent court hearing determined that Beau should not be allowed back into his owner's care and that he should be destroyed.

A FINAL COMMENT

Regarding Beau's routine management in kennels on both occasions, I see no reason whatsoever that anyone with a modicum of knowledge regarding dogs and their emotions could not have communicated with Beau as I did during the assessments. It is not rocket science.

In my opinion, there were two possibilities regarding kennel staff:

1. They did not have the prerequisite behavioural knowledge, in which case they should not be employed to care for long-term kennelled dogs.
2. The kennel staff did indeed have the knowledge but had been instructed not to use it.

I do not believe I am being overly cynical to suggest that a dog, having been seized as aggressive and dangerous, was being preserved to appear aggressive and dangerous in order to justify charges brought against the owner. There is no justification whatsoever for this approach. There was no consideration of Beau's mental welfare and how it impacted on his behaviour. To confine dogs in a kennel in such conditions can only be described as inhumane, and Beau is not alone to have suffered in this way.

4.   BAD HUMAN BEHAVIOUR

Buddy was a 4-year-old Staffordshire Bullterrier whose owner had been charged regarding an incident on 22nd January 2018. It had been alleged that, while dangerously out of control in a private place, Buddy had caused injury.

I already knew from documentation enough detail of the events of the evening in question to conclude that if Buddy had indeed bitten, it could hardly be considered to be 'all his fault' by any stretch of the imagination. A summary of the case was that Buddy first bit the hand of the owner's sister on her entry into the property, then jumped up and bit her boyfriend twice during subsequent arguments between them and between her and her sister. The exact sequence of events, over the course of two hours, was disputed but the consumption of alcohol by all concerned was mentioned, as well as the smashing of a plate on the floor, in Buddy's presence.

Additional contributory factors were identified via questionnaire and during my assessment at home.

BUDDY'S HISTORY

Buddy had been acquired in November 2017 as a 3-year-old dog, following an advert on Facebook. His previous owner could no longer have the dog in his flat owing to council restrictions. His microchip number was already registered to a dog rescue charity, indicating that the dog had already been relinquished to them at some unknown point in his life. There was also a record that Buddy had been owned for only two weeks by a female who 'couldn't cope' with him. Even without any further details, I realised that Buddy's history seemed to have been somewhat haphazard.

He now lived in the company of another Staffordshire Bullterrier dog called Diego and had been neutered under the auspices of the rescue society.

He was accepted to be a very excitable dog in greetings and his owner had been trying to deal with his overenthusiastic welcome of visitors. This had entailed trying to get him to sit, instead of jumping up, to 'bring his blanket' on which he was known to suckle and, since the incident, confining him in an indoor crate to allow him to calm down before release.

He was taken out twice a day in the company of his companion dog when there had never been any reported incidents. He could be safely let off lead and had a good recall.

DURING THE ASSESSMENT IN NOVEMBER 2018

On this occasion I was accompanied and assisted by my son, Linden. Upon our arrival at the house, Buddy's owner had obviously forgotten my instructions which were to place Buddy in his crate as she would routinely with any other previously unknown visitors to the house. I therefore saw immediately the worst excesses of Buddy's greeting behaviour when free.

The door was opened by the owner with the two dogs shut inside the living room. Once the front door was shut, she opened the living room door at which point both dogs jumped up vigorously at me. The companion dog simply leapt up into the air in my direction, whereas Buddy made many attempts to mouth my hands and clothing. Although these could not be described as 'bites', I could easily understand the potential for alarm and accidental injury or damage. Upon being restrained by the collar, he mouthed more vigorously in frustration but, once released, he obeyed a 'sit' command from me. Although his owner's commands, such as to 'calm down' or 'get down', had been ignored thus far, on being instructed by her to fetch 'blanket', Buddy picked up some bedding on the floor and stayed chewing at it.

In many ways, I had already seen enough of Buddy's behaviour to explain the beginning of the cascade of incidents as described in January 2018. However, I knew that, in addition to testing his responses in various contexts known to elicit aggression (such as vet examination and food guarding), the owner (and court) would have to understand that his behavioural prognosis would depend on improving his self-control, his trainability and the correction of some of the very common misunderstandings and mistakes owners make in communicating with their dogs. I therefore interspersed my assessment with training advice to improve his owner's control of Buddy specifically but also later to include the companion dog, who was equally excitable in greetings.

When I then asked for Buddy to be put on his normal lead, somewhat surprisingly, given his behaviour up to this point, he calmed down at the sight of his lead and remained standing with a gently wagging tail, whereas the majority of dogs might be expected to become excited.

COMMENTS AND CONCLUSIONS FROM MY REPORT

Buddy showed no aggression towards me or my assistant throughout the assessment. I accepted that his overly exuberant greeting behaviour and his response to frustration could, however, be alarming and result in accidental damage.

I explained that jumping up is part of normal canine greeting behaviour, as puppies do to their dam while in the litter. It is first rewarded by the dam allowing suckling and then, as the puppies grow older, negatively punished by the dam simply walking away. It is however retained in the canine repertoire as an appeasing part of greeting. Paradoxically, if paid attention or human anger results from jumping up, rather than being ignored, jumping up will get worse, as evidently it had in Buddy. Although his full history was not known, his suckling on a blanket as an adult might indicate lack of maternal care and appropriate early learning.

I believed the initial incident, where it was alleged that he nipped the hand of the owner's sister, to be the result of this exuberant greeting behaviour, as he displayed towards me. I did not believe he had any aggressive intent and, in the event itself, did not cause any injury.

It was stated that several arguments, some appearing to have been quite violent, transpired over the course of two hours for various reasons. The first began with the sister's annoyance at Buddy jumping up at her and later trying to grab her take-away food, at which point a plate was smashed. It is well recognised that dogs become distressed by human argument, all the more so if it is fuelled by alcohol. It is also known that, while arguing, the combatants do not tend to notice any early signs of canine unease or distress, and it is not uncommon in the cases I have seen that dogs will eventually have to nip or bite in order to stop human violence. **Paradoxically, therefore, a bite is intended to restore harmony rather than prolong it and in my experience, once driven to bite, a dog's actions are extremely effective in having the desired result and bringing inter-human conflict to an end.**

It is possible that the bites to the sister's boyfriend were in defence of the owner, but just as likely they were simply the result of the continuing conflict around Buddy and his perception of the male as an aggressor. A second bite inflicted was without doubt the result of his, or those around him, ignoring Buddy's first efforts at restoring peace.

Either way, I did not believe Buddy's actions were in any way evidence of a dangerous dog, rather the result of **intolerably bad human behaviour** while in his presence. He was an affectionate and highly trainable animal who bore no animosity towards people whatsoever. His propensity for jumping up was a training issue which, as demonstrated during my assessment, was likely to be successfully controlled if training were to be carried out consistently and clearly from his perspective.

A final, rather pointed comment was to express my surprise that police time and money had been spent on this case when, rather than prosecution for an allegedly dangerous dog, **all that was needed was acceptable human behaviour and a little dog training**. This dog owner, as a great number of others, was in need of advice as to how best to control Buddy's jumping up (by encouraging calm behaviour during greeting) but that this had to be accompanied by a full understanding of how human conflict can be a trigger for aggression in any dog.

5.   REDIRECTED AGGRESSION

Enzo was a 5½-year-old male neutered Staffordshire Bullterrier when, on 12th December 2018 he was alleged to have injured a 10-year-old boy. His owner was duly charged with allowing him to be dangerously out of control in a public place. A summary of the case in documentation received prior to my assessment revealed that Enzo was being walked by his owner in a park close to his home. The boy was playing football with a friend on one of the nearby football pitches. Enzo was let off lead to play with one dog and then a second younger Whippet dog joined in. Rather than following their owners, the Whippet, followed by Enzo, ran towards the football pitches. It was asserted by his owner that Enzo ran straight for the football, when the bites to the boy's leg occurred.

Enzo's owner, as well as the friend's father attempted to pull Enzo off the boy's leg and to pry his jaws apart. Once he had let go, and Enzo was restrained by her, the owner waited for the police to arrive. Enzo was then seized and had been in police custody for six months by the time of my assessment. By all accounts, including that of the boy himself, Enzo's owner was shocked and very distressed by what had happened. She expressed extreme remorse in her interview.

Enzo's routine history (stating that, apart from the occasional squabble with a companion dog, there had been no indication of aggression towards people or other dogs) was not received until after the assessment was carried out. But I was informed by police notes and also by his owner's police interview that, when rehomed at the age of 14 months, he already seemed to have an obsession with footballs and had in the past 'nipped ankles'.

THE ASSESSMENT

Apart from a little wriggling on examination of his ears, Enzo showed no aggression or inclination to bite throughout the assessment, despite its provocations. Rather he was an affectionate and extremely tolerant dog of human handling and intervention. He also showed no untoward behaviour to other dogs.

The following is a description of his specific responses during **toy-directed activity or play behaviour,** when it was anticipated that Enzo might be highly aroused by such objects, owing not only to his breed type but also his previous history. I attached a long line to his collar to give him more freedom than a training lead, in order to mimic, as closely as possible under the circumstances, an off-lead state.

> I first offered him a ball on a rope toy and tried to interest him in play with it. In complete opposition to the reaction of many dogs of his type in my experience, he initially showed no inclination to chase or jump up for it. After some encouragement, he engaged rather half-heartedly in a tug-of-war but let go when asked and sat on command. He then lost interest.

> I offered a rope tug toy, with which many dogs are encouraged (and therefore come to expect) to engage in a 'tug-of-war' with people, and then a tennis ball, again an item of interest for many dogs. Enzo showed no interest whatsoever in either object.

> Finally, with my assistant holding the long line, I offered Enzo a football which I kicked towards him. His demeanour changed entirely to want to hold the ball with his paws and bite at the sides to pick it up. As I kicked at it and tried to pull the ball out of his mouth, he growled loudly. I did not however interpret this as a defensive growl indicating a threat to bite if I continued, but a 'play growl' exhibited by many dogs, particularly, for example, in the Rottweiler breed. Although he jumped up at me as I continued to hold it, he let go almost immediately and was responsive to a sit command to have the ball returned to him. Although he tried to pounce on the ball if I approached to take it from him, he was easily deflected into a 'sit/stay', again to be allowed to have the ball again as a reward. I kicked at the ball multiple times while he had it in his mouth and again I took hold of it, with a food reward for letting it go. While he was holding the ball, I could handle him all over with no aggression shown.

As I repeated these simple exercises, Enzo learnt quickly that doing as I asked predicted a food reward as well as getting the ball returned to him, and he became more willing to let the ball go. It soon got to the point where, rather than chase after the ball, he had voluntarily come to me instead to sit and be rewarded. This preferred behaviour had continued even when I had again kicked the ball around.

COMMENTS ON THE ASSESSMENT

Enzo had showed an unusual intensity of play specifically directed towards footballs and, equally unusually, marked lack of interest in other commonly used dog toys.

I strongly recommended that if the court were to watch nothing else on the video recording of the assessment, they watch this section. It demonstrated quite clearly the highly unusual distinction this particular dog had in his mind between general dog toys and footballs, and the consequent dramatic difference in his expressed behaviour when exposed to them. It also showed how such behaviour could be managed and mentally controlled, if consistent behaviour modification and training techniques were to be used.

His owner related that this obsession with footballs had been an on-going issue throughout her ownership. The implication was that Enzo had been actively encouraged to play and chase footballs as a young dog <u>before</u> being rehomed by her and associated this item with human company and attention. An apparently harmless pastime had now had very unfortunate results.

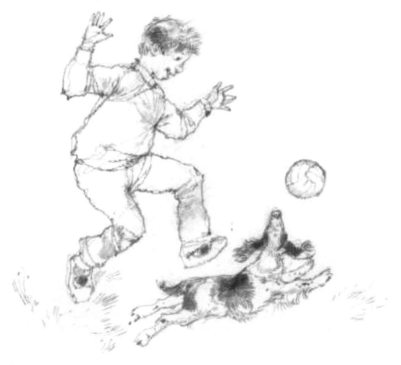

Illustration by Victor Ambrus.

I did not believe that Enzo bore any animosity towards the boy nor had any intention at all to bite him. The bites were, in my opinion, an example of **redirected aggression** in that the true target for Enzo was the ball, but that the boy's leg had simply got in the way. The arousal of previous play and chase with other dogs may have predisposed Enzo to being unable to think clearly at the time, in addition to the intense stimulus of the football itself.

The boy's statement indicated that his foot was bitten first, as would be the case if it was in the way of the ball. Enzo was then alleged to have bitten the upper leg, by which time the boy had obviously reacted in pain and had been attempting to kick Enzo away. This may well have then triggered the second bite. Enzo's owner also tried to pull Enzo away. Although these were of course perfectly normal and understandable reactions, they were unfortunately likely to have increased the intensity of Enzo's behaviour and grip, and thereby worsen any injury.

CONCLUSIONS AND RECOMMENDATIONS

To prevent any recurrence of the incident, I felt that ensuring future control had to be two-fold:

a.   physically controlling Enzo to ensure prevention
b.   using behaviour modification and training techniques to control his decisions and counter his football obsession

If on lead, I believed Enzo did not need muzzling, showing as he did no animosity to people or other dogs.

If allowed off lead and there was any risk of encountering football play, then Enzo should be muzzled, as demonstrated. However, I recommended that he should be kept on a long line, as I did, to allow some freedom but also to ensure that he could be physically held back from running off if needed.

No specific attempts had been made by his owner to alter Enzo's view of footballs. In the future, it was strongly recommended a qualified behaviourist was found to work with him along the lines demonstrated in my assessment. He also needed improved recall training in the presence of other dogs. While his intentions towards other people and dogs were entirely friendly, the consequences of lack of reliable recall from play were frequently very serious.

Enzo was allowed to return home after the court hearing and his owner received a fine and conditional discharge. The conditions were that he should be kept on lead and muzzled at all times in public and be excluded from entering the park containing football pitches. Yet again, physical restrictions only were relied upon to provide preventative control in the future and the opportunity for public education was missed.

6.   INAPPROPRIATE GREETING BEHAVIOUR AND MISDIRECTED PLAY

Bella, a 3½-year-old unneutered female Staffordshire Bullterrier cross, was being walked by her female owner in a local park. In the park there was a fenced grassy enclosure used by many dog walkers. Although the enclosure was gated, it was not secure as the gate could swing open freely. Bella was routinely walked on a fixed or extending lead owing to her propensity for chasing cats but was allowed off lead in the enclosure as she got on well with people and other dogs.

On this occasion, Bella slipped out of the gate and ran towards a group of children who were accompanied by an aunt. Despite Bella's owner's instructions not to run, one child ran away at her approach and it was alleged that Bella had chased her and at some point, the child had fallen over. It was also alleged that Bella had bitten the child's arm and clothes, including a scarf the child was wearing. Meanwhile, the aunt had attempted to pull her niece away from Bella.

As a result, Bella's owner was charged under the Dangerous Dogs Act with allowing a dog to become dangerously out of control and, while so out of control, to injure a person. Bella was, however, not taken into custody nor were there any control stipulations. I was therefore able to assess Bella at home with her owner and walk her outside the house to the nearby site of the incident in the normal way. My initial instructions were to assess Bella's behaviour and how it may have contributed to the incident, ultimately to give an opinion as to whether Bella was 'dangerous' and a risk to public safety.

THE ASSESSMENT

Upon my arrival at her home, Bella proved to be excitable and exuberant, but entirely friendly and non-aggressive. She allowed petting and handling straight away and did not present any threat to either me or to my assistant. She had a tendency to jump up in greeting as had been acknowledged in the pre-assessment questionnaire and was evidently a very appeasing dog, shown by laying her ears back, pawing and rolling on her back, as well as jumping up. I was informed that she sometimes passed a little urine when greeting visitors (so-called 'submissive urination', extra evidence of her wish to appease). In view of Bella's excitable nature, I interspersed my assessment of Bella with behaviour advice designed to calm Bella down and reduce her need to jump up.

Bella's owner's brother and young niece then arrived at the apartment un-announced. Bella became very excited in greeting them and proceeded to jump up vigorously. **While so doing, she removed a bobble hat from the child's head**. Although this caused some consternation at the time, it was, as luck would have it, extremely informative as to what may have happened on the day of the incident. I gave advice how best to deal with this essentially playful canine behaviour and stressed that this must not involve getting angry, chasing Bella or trying to pull things out of her mouth. All of these actions would simply encourage more grab-bing and stealing in order to engage companions in a chase and/or tug-of-war game.

At no point did Bella show any hint of aggression, simply exuberant playfulness. She readily dropped the hat in exchange for food and a more appropriate dog toy. It was, however, evident how readily she would have engaged a tug-of-war game had I allowed it. I also advised the young girl not to squeal or push Bella away as this would simply encourage more jumping up and instead to remain quiet, fold her arms and turn her body away.

Once we went outside, Bella showed herself to be very sociable, wanting to approach and greet all people we passed. She immediately allowed and enjoyed petting and stroking by a passer-by. She showed a tendency to jump up towards them but remained with a very friendly demeanour. I continued to demonstrate to her owner how easily Bella could be asked to sit as an appropriate and pleasant control measure.

We walked to the enclosed grass area described in the statements, which was used routinely by other dog walkers and where Bella was exercising off lead just prior to the incident. I confirmed that the gate to the area pulled shut but did not have a catch or fastening. I was also shown the block paving walkway and sloped side on which the children were playing when Bella approached them.

I then transferred Bella onto a long line to more closely resemble complete freedom as she inadvertently had on the day of the incident. I deliberately excited Bella several times at the site, encouraging her to jump up and to grab a scarf around my neck. I also provoked her with a toy on a rope and engaged in a tug-of-war game with her. Despite her arousal, she responded instantly to a sit command. She also allowed me to forcefully remove both toy and scarf from her mouth, to forcefully restrain her and handle all parts of her body. She showed no aggression at any point. I continued to instruct her owner how best to call Bella to her and ask her to sit as well as showing how easily Bella would drop one toy in exchange for another.

Although there was plenty of evidence of Bella's highly sociable and friendly nature towards people, I advised her owner that allowing Bella routinely to approach all passers-by whenever she wanted to had created an expectation in Bella that this was the automatic and accepted thing to do. For future training, it would be better to intersperse some sociable interactions with being called back to her owner and asked to sit in exchange for a food reward. It was of particular importance to do this if Bella came across those who may be afraid of dogs. This control measure was demonstrated several times during our return home, during which both dog and owner were responding briskly and appropriately.

The young niece was also delighted in her newfound ability to ask Bella to sit for a toy rather than jump up at her.

OPINION GIVEN AND CONCLUSIONS

I found that Bella could not be described as a dangerous dog by any stretch of the imagination.

In my first court report, I proposed that the incident had been the accidental result of the following behavioural characteristics, which had been clearly shown and confirmed during my assessment.

- An extremely sociable and friendly nature towards people, resulting in the routine investigation of social contacts outside the house
- Extremely exuberant playfulness

- Accidentally reinforced jumping up in greeting
- A high level of toy-directed play and enjoyment of tug-of-war games
- Insufficient rehearsal and use of already-known obedience commands

I acknowledged that these features could result in accidental injury but had found no evidence of Bella trying to, or mistakenly biting, arms or clothing when aroused, as alleged. The only proviso was that a scarf might be mistaken for a tug toy.

The second court hearing was to be a so-called Newton Hearing. These are held when certain relevant facts are disputed and have to be established before the case is heard. On this occasion, whether Bella had bitten as alleged was pertinent to any judgement made against her owner. The court had therefore instructed that the prosecution must supply me with witness statements and colour photographs of the injuries sustained which had been missing from the original bundle. I was duly instructed to provide an addendum report giving my opinion as to whether there was any evidence to support the allegation that Bella had bitten, given the nature of the injuries as depicted.

Once I received the photographs I could clearly see that the injury to the child's arm was not consistent with a bite and, having seen where the incident took place, was far more likely to have been a graze suffered when falling onto the sloped, paved surface. This I found was described as a hill in the transcript of the child's interview. She had also suffered an injury to her neck. The photographic evidence showed a horizontal contusion with a distinct pattern such as might be inflicted by tightening of a thin rope or by a scarf with a piped edge.

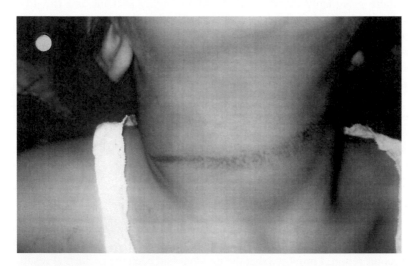

I had seen during the assessment how easily Bella could be encouraged to jump for a scarf and use it as a tug toy and the fact that the child had been pulled away bodily by her aunt was confirmed by her interview.

I therefore concluded that Bella tugging on the child's scarf in one direction, and the aunt pulling the child bodily in the other, had resulted in a 'rope burn' around the child's neck.

I acknowledged that the aunt's actions had been understandable in the heat of the moment but were ill-advised and would have contributed to the severity of the injury.

I confirmed my previous opinion that this additional evidence did not indicate any intention to harm on Bella's part and that neither injury was consistent with a bite. Her actions were the result of exuberant and inappropriate play behaviour and the injuries as depicted supported this interpretation.

Around about the same time as this case, I came across a news item regarding a visit by Camilla, Duchess of Cornwall, to a police dog training establishment. During this visit, an incident was caught on camera when a young German Shepherd jumped up and grabbed the scarf she was wearing around her neck. This was simply reported as an amusing tale rather than as evidence of a dangerous dog. But why should this be? Because Camilla's reaction had been simply to laugh rather than panic.

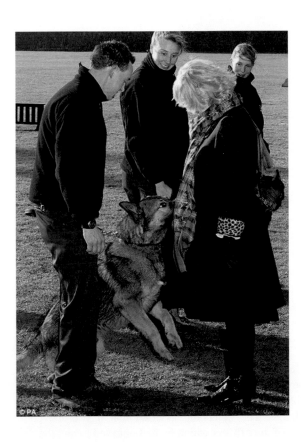

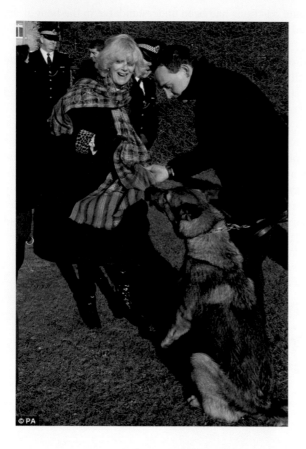

7. CONFLICT WITH POLICE

The owner of a dog called Rolex had been charged under Section 1 of the Dangerous Dogs Act with being the owner of a Pitbull terrier type dog. He had also been charged with obstructing a constable in the execution of his duty. I was instructed to assess Rolex primarily to give an opinion as to whether his conformation complied with the ADBA standard for the Pitbull terrier (see Chapter 11 Dangerous Dogs Act). I was also to assess the dog's behaviour and how it might relate to the incident as described.

THE INCIDENT

The defendant was seen walking a dog which was suspected by police officers driving past to be of the Pitbull type. They then left their van and confronted him, demanding that he hand over his dog. It was alleged that he had been obstructive in being unwilling to do this, hence the second charge. The defendant asserted that it was the confrontational and aggressive attitude of the officers which he had objected to and that he had had no reason previously to suspect that his dog was a Pitbull type. It was also alleged that Rolex scratched one of the officers during the confrontation.

Uniquely, the incident had in part been captured on video by builders working on the opposite side of the road so that I could take this evidence into account as well as the normal witness statements and the results of my behaviour assessment.

THE ASSESSMENT

This was carried out five months after Rolex's seizure. As I was not to be allowed into his holding kennels, he was transported to a mutually agreed farm premises to be assessed. Rolex was eminently friendly when I removed him from the transport van. First of all I examined him to determine the degree to which his anatomy and, to a lesser degree, his behaviour, conformed to the ADBA breed standard. It involved taking several measurements to accurately determine the ratios between certain skeletal features specified in the breed standard and giving a subjective opinion on others, such as the set of the teeth. This examination is of itself a test of a dog's tolerance involving enforced restraint and intimate handling. It cannot be tolerated by some dogs, when a purely visual assessment has to be made at the time and later from the video recording and photographs.

I then carried out the normal gamut of behavioural tests, including veterinary examination, grooming, toy-directed play and food guarding. He remained tolerant and friendly throughout.

In this case, it was particularly important to gauge his behavioural response to human conflict and argument. Rolex had been taken from his owner on the street in a situation of human confrontation. It was therefore necessary to test his response to a simulated physical argument between me and Rod, which included shouting and much pushing and shoving. For safety's sake, I fitted Rolex with a muzzle beforehand which he immediately tolerated. During our 'argument', Rolex became aroused, jumping up vigorously towards both of us. He showed no aggression, however, and calmed down the instant we did. I could immediately remove the muzzle, after which he took food gently from both of us and sat on command.

Methodology for the assessment of Pitbull type dogs (DDA Section 1)

All my assessments are video recorded as well as detailed photographs taken. I am therefore able to assess any dog visually by later review of the recording and photographs as well as directly at the time, allowing me to confirm my opinion as to their overall appearance and general anatomical conformation to the ADBA breed standard for the pure-bred Pitbull terrier, as well as behavioural attributes as required, such as demeanour and attitude.

I intend to take all measurements required to thoroughly assess the dogs' bodily conformation to this standard. It must be emphasised that it is not the objective measurements *per se* which are of relevance, as the Pitbull breed and therefore type may differ quite widely in size and weight, but the ratios that exist between certain parts of the body. These ratios, in my opinion, can only be accurately determined by measurement of the specified body parts in relation to each other. I routinely use a large caliper to measure, for example, the shoulder and cheek width, a small TB testing caliper to measure skin thickness, and both fabric and rigid metal tape measures for other features, such as the height and length of the dog. All measurements are recorded at the time, copies of which are contained in the Addenda.

The analysis is based upon the American Dog Breeders Association standard for the pure-bred Pitbull terrier as detailed in the Pitbull Gazette magazine article of 1977 (written by Ralph Greenwood). **It must be stressed that this standard was only ever intended to be used by experienced judges to judge pure-bred dogs in the show ring and to award points for how closely they matched it.** It was never intended to be used to judge the degree of conformity of a cross-bred dog or mongrel to the standard for a pure-bred animal.

The ADBA show standard for the Pitbull terrier allows 10 out of 100 points to be awarded for a dog's demeanour or attitude. This is defined, confirmed by the ADBA, as being: confident and alert; interested in things around them; not threatened by their environment; and gentle and non-aggressive to loved ones. **Man-aggression in any form is considered to be an absolute fault.** It is considered acceptable that a dog may exhibit aggression towards other dogs, given the purpose for which the dog was originally selected and bred. In order to fulfill its function as a fighting dog, a Pitbull terrier was also required to show 'gameness', or tenacity in persisting in any given behaviour. I use object (toy)-directed 'play' to assess: desire to grab and hold; persistence or tenacity; athleticism and agility; accuracy; and tolerance of frustration. These behavioural features are also required as part of the determination of the prognosis for dogs as regards the risk they may or may not pose in the future.

CONCLUSIONS AND COMMENTS

THE TYPE ASSESSMENT

I found Rolex to be a 'borderline' dog in that he carried 64% of 'Pitbull type' features and felt that a court was very likely to find him of the Pitbull type. Personally, I have used two-thirds of features (66%) as a benchmark for determining type. Such dogs begin to resemble the real thing sufficiently to fool the casual onlooker, but I doubt, however, that they would pass muster as a pure-bred Pitbull terrier to an experienced judge's eye in an American show ring. In any event, one sincerely hopes that such pseudo-scientific nonsense linking appearance with dangerousness will be soon consigned to the history books.

THE BEHAVIOUR ASSESSMENT WITH PARTICULAR REFERENCE TO THE CIRCUMSTANCES OF HIS SEIZURE

Regarding his behaviour, Rolex showed no aggression whatsoever throughout my assessment, despite its many provocations. It is a paradox that my assessment of him as a friendly, exuberant, tolerant and playful dog contributed to his designation as a dangerous Pitbull type.

Despite his excitement and exuberance, he showed himself to be gentle with his mouth and readily responsive to obedience training.

I had been instructed specifically to comment on the video clip supplied and Rolex's behaviour at the time, with reference to my assessment of him. My observations and comments taken directly from my report were as follows:

- The video clip begins with his owner still having Rolex's lead in his hand and a female police officer appears to be asking him to relinquish his dog. As might be understandable, his owner is remonstrating with the police in order to protect his dog.
- Very shortly, his owner releases the lead to her, which is then passed to one of two male police officers. I am unable to ascertain from the statements which one. Rolex is jumping up in an excited manner, obviously distressed by what is going on, but in my view is showing no aggression whatsoever.
- The officers between them then tether Rolex to a parking restriction post against which a bicycle is propped. During this, Rolex jumps up at one of the officers, resulting in his cap falling off. In addition, the bicycle is knocked over. Despite the commotion, Rolex's observed behaviour is in no way aggressive.
- Rolex is then left to observe his owner, in his eyes, being accosted by three, later four, strangers (in other words, the officers attempting to handcuff and arrest his owner) and be unable to intervene. He therefore begins to bark. Intent on the 'execution of their duty', the arresting officers seem oblivious to the presence of several passers-by who could, if Rolex had indeed presented a danger, been put at risk from an unattended tethered dog.
- In my opinion, at no time does Rolex display aggression but rather behaviour consistent with a confused and distressed, but human-friendly, dog attempting to intervene in what was perceived as conflict and violence. The behaviour shown in this video clip is consistent with that seen during my assessment, when he jumped up vigorously as a result of simulated human conflict.

Jumping up is part of a repertoire of canine appeasement behaviour most frequently displayed during greetings. It is of itself entirely devoid of any aggressive intent. The intention of all appeasement behaviour is to result in a reduction of threat and restore harmony. Although jumping up may be potentially alarming, it is frequently inadvertently rewarded and reinforced by human response, in the form of petting and attention. In the absence of an expected response, jumping up, as any other behaviour, canine or human, may become more pronounced, which appears to have happened here.

FURTHER COMMENTS MADE

With respect to the officers involved, the video clip demonstrated clearly the lack of suitable training of officers when dealing with a person accompanied by their dog. There is much scientific evidence of the mutually beneficial bond between humans and dogs which has evolved over many thousands of years, and, whether an individual is aware of it or not, the perception is that a dog is akin to close friend or a child. Whatever one perceives their 'duty' to be, one cannot simply approach and forcefully remove an animal, which could be perceived as either, without expecting vigorous objection.

I had no doubt that Rolex was in no way an aggressive dog and, should the court find that he is of the Pitbull type, was entirely suitable to be allowed onto the Exempt Register.

OUTCOME

Rolex was found to be a Pitbull type by the Court but allowed to return home under the conditions of the Exempt Register. His owner was found *not guilty* of the charge of obstructing a constable in the execution of his duty.

SUMMARY

I hope that this chapter has given the reader a flavour of what I have found is entailed in assessing the temperament and behaviour of dogs the law deems to be, rightly or wrongly, dangerous. While being critical of the legislation as it stands, I am very conscious of the need to have some means of determining the real risk an individual dog poses and the obligation one has to be as honest and as accurate as possible, taking all current knowledge into account.

There seems still to be dissent and debate in this and in other countries regarding why and how behavioural assessments should be conducted. My chapter in 'Dog Bites' (Shepherd 2017) is I believe a first – a personal attempt to set down a methodology which takes all available information about a dog into account to create a prognosis for the future as well as ensuring that the assessment itself does not cause behavioural damage. The one variable that is almost impossible to quantify is that of future human behaviour.

There is an obvious need for the creation and recognition of the field of **forensic clinical animal behaviour**, in particular as it relates to dogs. It must be emphasised that the word 'forensic' does not, as is often assumed, mean solely the study of corpses or their dissection for diagnostic purposes to determine the cause of death. Instead, it refers to any field which may be 'relating to, used in, or connected with a court of law' (Cooper and Cooper 2018). This particular article focuses on veterinary forensic medicine and stresses how this may differ from routine diagnosis and treatment, in particular the need for 'strict adherence to protocols and standard procedures'. If the field of forensic clinical animal behaviour is to be taken seriously, it is therefore surely first necessary for there to be 'protocols and standard procedures' available to be adhered to?

Just as this book has the intention of encouraging more veterinary surgeons to become involved in the behaviour of dogs as it applies to their day-to-day work and commitment to animal welfare, I would further the plea for more veterinary surgeons to pick up the cudgel of legal work. It is indeed stressful, involves routine attempts by the opposition to undermine one's expertise and is not for the faint-hearted. But having the opportunity to successfully explain the Ladder of Aggression to a Magistrates' bench or a jury is immensely satisfying. As for the gratitude expressed by a client whose dog has been saved from a needless death, it easily equates to, or even exceeds, that received following life-saving surgery.

13 The dilemma dogs face

This is not strictly speaking a legal case which came to court but involved legal requirements. It is an illustration of how unrealistic expectations are made of dogs. What happens when the requirements of society are in conflict with that of the owner and a dog's breed-related behaviour? How can we reconcile them?

A 3½-year-old entire male German Shepherd dog named 'Reece' was owned by a traveller family residing at the time in Fakenham Temporary Stopping Place, A148, Holt Road, Fakenham Norfolk (permission granted for all details to be published).

I was asked by the Equality and Diversity Manager at Community and Environmental Services, Norfolk County Council, to assess Reece as regards his behaviour, the training and management protocols the owner had in place and, consequently, any risk he may or may not pose to the general public. This was in light of an up and coming move to the more permanent traveller site of The Splashes, Castle Acre Road, Swaffham where his owner very much hoped to be able to stay with Reece and her extended family. It seemed as if concerns regarding the behaviour of Reece expressed by council workers and the risk he might pose would preclude this move.

The following information was given in the pre-assessment questionnaire:

Reece had been obtained in March 2018 from a family who had used him as a protection dog for a collection of vintage vehicles. His history before then, or means of upbringing, was not known but I was led to believe that he had never been an indoor dog or considered to be a pet.

Reece was registered for veterinary treatment at a Veterinary Centre in Saxilby, Lincoln. Re-registration at a new surgery was planned if and when permission was granted for the hoped-for move to Swaffham.

Reece had had one-to-one training sessions with a trainer who had advised re-straining Reece on a choke chain and using coercive methods. Video footage of certain such training sessions had been supplied to me.

Reece was considered to be a playful and obedient dog who was tolerant of all people of any age or sex as long as they were known to him. He lived routinely with several other small dogs, a cat and several birds to which he had never shown any aggression. He was therefore able to be left free to roam within the enclosed Stopping Place unless anyone he did not know was expected.

He was known to bark vigorously at anyone he did not know when chained at the gate and 'on duty'. **This was what was required of him as a protective deterrent, when he was considered by the family to be 'working'.**

Reece was never routinely taken inside any trailer or caravan and had a kennel with bedding when chained outside close to the entrance gate. Although not yet erected on this site, owing to its supposedly temporary nature, and stored elsewhere, his alternative accommodation was a standard roofed secure kennel unit, incorporating both sleeping and run areas. If it were exceptionally cold, as it was on the day of my assessment, he was allowed into and contained in a horsebox.

When taken out in town, Reece was always kept on lead and might wear a muzzle, if in close proximity to people. This was to ward off those who might have the desire to approach and pet him (as people unfortunately and ill-advisedly might have the tendency to do to a handsome dog) as much as to ameliorate risk.

When walked in fields and woods outside the enclosure, Reece was routinely walked on a horse lunge line so that he could be given more freedom. Although people were rarely encountered, he showed no apprehension of or untoward behaviour towards anyone he did meet.

There was no record of any untoward incident involving this dog since in the possession of his owner.

THE ASSESSMENT

I visited the Stopping Place in Fakenham in January 2019. Rod and I were accompanied by a country-wide Gypsy, Roma and Traveller Liaison Officer who was extremely helpful in facilitating introductions owing to the family's understandable mistrust of outside interference and the prospect of video recording. They were assured that the recording would not include any vehicle registration numbers, nor of anyone, including children, without their expressed permission.

Upon our arrival, Reece was secured in a horsebox, as was the routine in any event, owing to the subzero temperatures. I spent some time gathering more information about Reece, his management and training and acquainting myself with the family. Present were Ryalla Duffy, Brittania, Verity, Eliza and Absolom (all adult), as well as others of the extended family, at various times.

After some 30 minutes, I asked Ryalla to bring Reece out of the horsebox so that we could first observe and then meet him. There were a number of other small dogs, restrained on a tether or in cages, who barked continuously while we were there. She walked him around first of all on a training lead, then a lunge line, attached to a thin rope check collar, keeping him under tight restraint. She demonstrated how he would sit by her side.

He was first of all unperturbed by our presence but soon became alarmed by the sight of Rod with the video camera and began to bark at him. He also barked at Absolom, standing next to us, who, although familiar to him, was, I was told, wearing an unaccustomed coat. Of necessity some of the earlier parts of the filming were taken by zooming in from a distance.

He continued to bark at me as I approached him and Ryalla, although with wagging tail which showed emotional conflict. Ryalla then had more difficulty in making him sit and he would not take thrown food titbits from me owing to his aroused emotional state. He was also still barking at Absolom, who had no fear in walking up to Reece to pet him. If allowed more freedom on the lunge line, he continued to bark but voluntarily followed Ryalla as she moved away. He continued to bark at me even when I was sitting down to reduce perceived threat.

I had asked on arrival if any children were present on the site and if any of them would be happy to interact with Reece. A 10-year-old girl called Star volunteered. She watched Reece barking to begin with but a short while later showed no hesitation in approaching him.

Absolom then took charge of the lunge line, as he frequently walked Reece. Reece pulled towards Ryalla but was restrained and made to sit easily by him. Reece remained calmly sitting even with me in his close vicinity. I asked Ryalla to approach Reece and give him a piece of food, which he then ate, indicating that he was becoming more relaxed. Ryalla then put Reece back on the training lead. I asked her to attach it to the half-check collar already around his neck, rather than the rope choke collar and to try to be as relaxed as possible with him. Reece then performed a calm 'sit-stay' without barking. I concluded that the more freedom he was given, the less reason Reece had to feel defensive.

Ryalla then walked him round in front of Rod, so he was filming at close quarters. There was no barking. He was asked to sit easily and took food thrown by me towards him as a reward for sitting. He remained calm with gently wagging tail, until he got rather too close to me and then began barking again. He was easily led away by Ryalla.

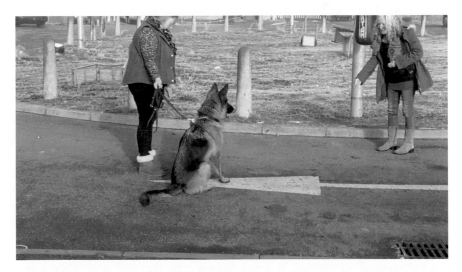

A few moments were then spent walking Reece around and intermittently asking him to sit. I explained that obedience exercises act as emotional stabilisers, in that the part of the brain involved in 'obeying', (thinking about what had to be done and doing it) counteracted the reactive 'fight or flight' side when no guidance was given. As I was explaining this, Reece stood and sat calmly and eventually rolled over on his side to allow both Ryalla and Absolom to tickle his tummy. Absolom showed clearly how he could put his hand between Reece's teeth without being bitten.

We then walked out of the enclosure along a path towards neighbouring fields. Although alerting to me, Reece allowed me to walk past him on the path without barking and to walk alongside him. After a few moments, I asked Ryalla again to put him in a 'sit'. He then moved slightly towards me, and Ryalla, as she had done before, restrained him and told him to sit. I then asked her to relax and let him come to me. He simply took food gently from my hand.

We entered a field with horses belonging to the Duffy family. Reece was completely calm with no untoward reaction. Several times I asked Reece to come to me and to sit. He was thoroughly compliant and allowed me to stroke and fondle his head. No barking or aggression was shown. He also obeyed a 'lie down' command from me. As he was a little demanding, pawing at me for food, I demonstrated how to teach him he would get food only by being patient. Showing him a closed fist containing food, I only opened it when he pulled his head back or turned his head away from my hand. Thereafter I could still fondle his head and scratch all along his back with no reaction.

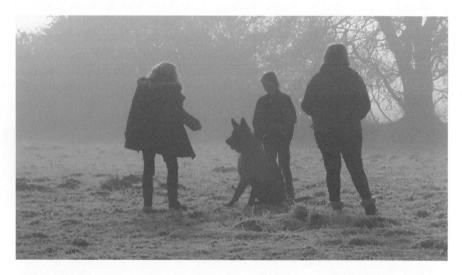

Shortly thereafter, Reece began barking, not in the direction of Rod and the camera but at Absolom who had appeared on the path. Star also came towards us and Ryalla handed her the lead to walk Reece, as she had done before. Even while Reece was barking, Star had no apprehension about petting and stroking Reece on the head.

On our return to the enclosed site, Reece was more alert to the barking around him but showed no wariness at being followed by the camera or when walking closely by my side. He sat both voluntarily and, when told, took food and allowed me to pet and stroke him as before.

We then spent some time discussing muzzle training. As I intended to examine him as a vet might and despite the progress he had shown with me as a 'normal' person, there was no guarantee this view would extend into the veterinary context. I therefore needed to muzzle him for safety reasons. I demonstrated a basket-type muzzle and showed how to associate wearing it with the delivery of food. Reece showed no objection to the muzzle being placed and continued to take food through the mesh.

I then scanned him for the presence of a microchip. Reece continued to allow me to fondle his head and ears while I was doing this and he remained calm throughout.

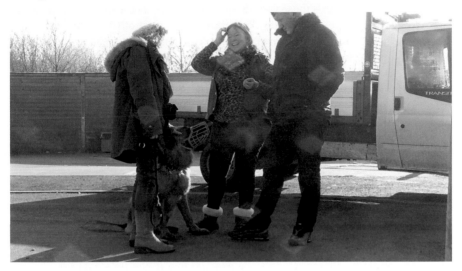

I then picked up a stethoscope in order to listen to his heart and lungs. In a response which took both Ryalla and me by surprise, he very suddenly reverted to his lunging and barking behaviour in my direction. Once I had put the stethoscope down out of sight, he tolerated my giving him food through the muzzle, but resumed barking shortly afterwards. This reaction, surprising as it was to begin with, was thoroughly explained by his previous veterinary experience, described below.

Reece was then walked around to allow him to relax, and he conveniently demonstrated how a dog is still able to drink (and of course pant) in such a muzzle by lapping up water from a puddle. I took the lead to walk him and he allowed me to pet him and massage his neck as he had before. He sat voluntarily by my side to be stroked and then lay down on his side as he had before in a completely relaxed manner.

Finally, Reece was put back on his chain, some 15 yards in length, at the gate. He immediately reverted to 'on guard' duty and ran to and fro, barking indiscriminately.

COMMENTS ON THE HISTORY, TRAINING AND ASSESSMENT OF REECE

Reece had never been intended to be a pet dog, expected instead to guard and protect against all comers, except for those he knew and was bonded to. He would therefore accept attention from those he knew and not necessarily from those he did not. It was not possible to comment specifically on his early upbringing or on how he was managed and treated, other than to say that it was likely he had been chained up and left to behave as Reece himself saw fit.

The German Shepherd is the breed of choice for police and military work, given the breed's reactivity, agility, trainability and perceived loyalty; in other words, being comfortable with and protective of those they know but wary of and potentially aggressive towards those they do not know. They are also very vocal dogs, using barking for a variety of reasons, but above all to alert others to the arrival of people, whether known or unknown, and as a means of expressing their own wariness and perception of threat.

Barking as a behaviour is unlikely to have been trained into any such dog generally and Reece specifically. In effect, wariness of strangers and barking as a means of warning may be the default canine behaviour in this breed. If a dog is expected to be friendly towards all strangers, implying being unafraid of them, then this must be taught from puppyhood in all dogs, particularly in breeds with a tendency to guard (in other words to be wary of strangers). If a dog is to become a protection dog, then this process of socialisation is simply left out.

Reece's one-to-one trainer was known for the training of protection dogs. He had given training advice as to how to control Reece in public, as could be seen in the video clip. It showed Reece sitting calmly, although alert, at Ryalla's side, but without a held lead, thus under mental control only. Ryalla was using kit that has been recommended by him, including the rope check/choke collar.

My assessment confirmed Reece to be exactly akin to the police dog of choice. He was trainable, in that he could learn new things very quickly; he was alert and reactive, perceiving and reacting to tiny changes in his environment, such as the coat change in Absolom and the presence of a stethoscope in my hand predicting veterinary attention; and 'protective' in that his propensity to vocalise and apparently threaten aggression served as a deterrent to intruders.

One has to differentiate between a dog barking apparently aggressively and a dog that means to bite. Barking, as did Reece, with wide open mouth showing all his teeth is a means dogs will use to deflect threat by appearing scary but achieves its purpose (from both canine and human perspectives) without being forced to bite. Dogs which do not tend to bark but deflect threat at very close quarters by biting with no prior warning, may be the more dangerous.

There was a distinct difference in Reece's demeanour towards me within the enclosure, when he viewed me as an intruder (hence a threat), and outside, when I was a normal person who did not present a threat. He allowed me to pet and stroke him, obeyed commands and took food gently from my hand. When I walked with him into the enclosure, he continued to be utterly tolerant of my presence and attention, having become familiar with me. He allowed me to scan him for a microchip but, at the time inexplicably, his demeanour changed once he perceived me as a vet. Shortly afterwards, however, he returned to his tolerant state. Once put back on his chain at the gate, it was remarkable how his behaviour changed to one of guarding and apparent protection. He was indeed a dog who, by virtue of environmental triggers rather than human training, knew exactly what to do, as any dog, when he needed to act in his own self-defence. His actions just happened to suit human requirements.

After my assessment of Reece, I obtained his veterinary records from when he needed to be seen for diarrhoea and an irritating rash on his belly in July 2018. He was taken to the surgery and muzzled in advance of the examination as a precaution by Ryalla's daughter, Britannia. The records described him as 'muzzled but aggressive' with no further information. Britannia had told me that, before he became 'stressed' (she recognised aggression as a symptom of stress in Reece), the attending veterinary surgeon attempted to force him to get onto a steel examination table. This is ill-advised for any large dog, much less one which has been presented muzzled and, almost without question, would not be attempted with a police dog. This unpleasant experience could well explain, in such an observant and reactive dog, the change in his demeanour once he saw a stethoscope in my hand.

ADDITIONAL BEHAVIOUR AND TRAINING ADVICE GIVEN

I was not altogether happy with the methods Ryalla had been using to encourage obedience in Reece. Some food had been used as rewards, but when on lead in public, reliance had been mainly upon the rope choke collar. As this functioned by applying an unpleasant choking sensation to the dog's neck, which was released when the dog obeyed, there was a danger that when the choke was applied, negative associations were made with other unintended features of the environment. This might include members of the public. Ryalla was not to be blamed for not realising this, as it is a common failing in all who use positive punishment as a training tool, including trainers themselves. If, however, it was intended that dogs should view strangers as a threat, in public as well as within a territory, then this technique may well have elicited the desired response.

I therefore advised that when outside the enclosed site in public, any correct response to the application of the choke collar, for example to sit, should be followed immediately with a food titbit. The effect of the collar would thereby be reinforced by the addition of food and would reduce the risk of negative associations being made with members of the public at large. I also advised that if Reece behaved well of his own volition, he should be rewarded with food. He would then tend to do more of what seemed to result in food, without the need for coercion in the first place.

Ryalla had however found, with which I entirely agreed, that Reece was very attentive to her movements (again as befitted the breed) and walking slowly, simply stopping if he pulled, and changing direction for him to follow her had been effective without having to apply the choke.

I also showed Ryalla how to make pleasant associations with the muzzle itself (by using it as a food dispenser) so that Reece looked forward to wearing it and it was considered normal to him. It is unfortunately common for dogs that may need muzzling in certain situations, for example for veterinary examination, that the muzzle comes to predict the emotion of fear and sensation of pain. He was also to be muzzled sometimes on the site itself and be cuddled by his family while wearing it to ensure that pleasant associations persisted.

When in town, and whether or not people were in close proximity or in crowds, I advised that the muzzle should be worn as a precaution, regardless of the admirable self- and owner control of Reece shown in the training video. One cannot guard too much against unforeseen events, as long as the muzzle itself does not trigger wariness. I did not feel it did, as shown in the assessment, and efforts had to be made to keep it that way.

Taking into account the need for Reece to behave protectively when inside the compound, I emphasised that this change in training him more positively in public would not affect his protective role. Barking at strangers was highly unlikely to have been deliberately trained. Barking as a behaviour is most commonly reinforced and perpetuated by changes in the environment itself, without owner interference. Passers-by and postmen, for example, are barked at and then routinely continue to pass by or retreat after delivery of letters. In the dog's eyes, his behaviour has been successful and therefore reinforced. I felt that there would be plenty of opportunity for Reece to rehearse barking in his current situation.

CONCLUSIONS

The aim of the Duffys, that of having a protective dog to act as a deterrent in the event of potential intruders, had to be reconciled with concerns of Norfolk County Council that the dog would be controlled and managed in such a way as to not present a danger to the public at large.

I was assured by Ryalla Duffy that, in all circumstances, Reece would either be on his chain by the gate; in his secure kennel once re-erected; be walked on lead/long line in the vicinity of the future compound; or in town, on lead and muzzled. In other words, he would either be confined or closely supervised and under full control.

It was indeed a tall order for a dog to be expected to behave as Reece did, friendly and tolerant one minute but on guard the next. In my heart of hearts, I would prefer for dogs not to be used in this way, including by the police, as I feel that we humans are taking advantage of a dog's innate apprehension and fear. This is inevitably accompanied by stress and emotional conflict in the dog.

However, I understood fully the reasons why Reece needed to be as he was, and I found him to be immensely suitable for this niche. It would be a very brave or very stupid intruder who would not be deterred by Reece at his most intimidating. I believed that the Duffy family were very understanding of his personality, body language and emotional needs and how much they depended on the results of this assessment. Reece's behaviour could not be allowed to jeopardise their move. I therefore believed that they would follow to the letter any conditions that may be placed on them regarding Reece, including the advice I had given.

My conclusion was that, under the conditions stated above, Reece, as far as could be envisaged with any dog, would not present a risk to the general public.

The Duffys were given the permission they needed to move to the permanent site.

Ryalla and I have since become friends. I have continued to receive updates about Reece and how he is behaving. My prediction that he was capable of fulfilling his dual role under the Duffy management has proved correct. This has been entirely due to Ryalla's complete understanding of the bigger picture and how Reece fitted into it.

I quote,

> 'Reece was a good boy at the weekend, worked very well. Some trespassers needed encouragement to move and he was very encouraging. He's been very good for settling things down at Swaffham as well, real game changer. Was offered very good money for him but he won't ever be for sale. Partners for life'.

Interestingly, it seems that his presence has also had a calming effect on the more unruly human elements of the new site, where Ryalla, through force of nature, has been accepted as undisputed Queen Bee.

> 'There were some issues on the site the other day and Reece did his job very very well. He knew exactly what he was doing as a deterrent and behaved impeccably. He is also wonderful round the small children. They play within reach and ignore him and he keeps a respectful distance and just watches with his head between his paws and rolls his eyes'. 😊

I asked for permission from Ryalla to include Reece's case here as all the elements of it are so relevant to the issues I have addressed in this book. At the most basic level, it was an opportunity, as in any consultation, to explain the common misunderstandings about how dogs learn and how we attempt to train them. But far more than this, the whole experience was a real eye-opener in terms of how our differing requirements of dogs can be reconciled and, moreover, how a dog can be central to bringing communities together. To begin with, I was mistrusted as an outsider – and the more I've learned about the prejudices that travellers are subjected to, the more I've understood they have good reason for this. Maybe it was initially thought that I was going to simply wade in with a superior attitude and a set of instructions on the basis that I knew better than they did.

But by focussing on Reece, a representative of a species laden with prejudices of its own, barriers seemed to fade away. His story is the perfect example of 'Zips Theory'. As long as we can agree about how a problem can be solved, we should not be judgemental about individual reasons why.

I'll leave the final words to Ryalla:

> Yes, it was such a success story and will continue to be so. Reece wasn't happy at Fakenham; the police were very aggressive and harassing and he picked up on all that. He likes it here on his hill under the shade of the pine trees, he has a good vantage point. He's loose all the time in the yard when I'm outside which is good for us both, and he has a good run each day.

> I'm looking at setting a new site up and implementing the management changes that the council here weren't able to do. None of the council staff here were experienced at effective site management and none of them had done any specific training but gone to the job from different roles. It's been wicked seeing the waste of money here and the total cost ineffectiveness. Residents have no respect for the management team and it's easy to see why. It's not rocket science. Firm but fair and then follow through and keep practising. Old habits can be changed with patience and persistence. Reece is

wonderful; we have a strong relationship as a team. We both think the others' safety and well-being are paramount. There's a good balance of work time, rest time and play time. It's amazing how dogs have empathy for our emotions.

I'll be leaving Swaffham soon to set up a new site from scratch and manage it. Reece is having a big run by the entrance and got fields all round for exercise. He makes everybody feel safe.

Reece is an integral part of our life: his mental, emotional and physical well-being is important. He needs fun and freedom to be happy, too. We are his family as much as he is ours. He likes going off in the camper that's his new delight. He flies like a bullet to get in and go for jollies. One of his strengths is visual and audio impact. It's daunting for uninvited visitors when he appears, and he never backs down. Yes, when we get settled you're very welcome to come and take tea, and we can have a good catch up.

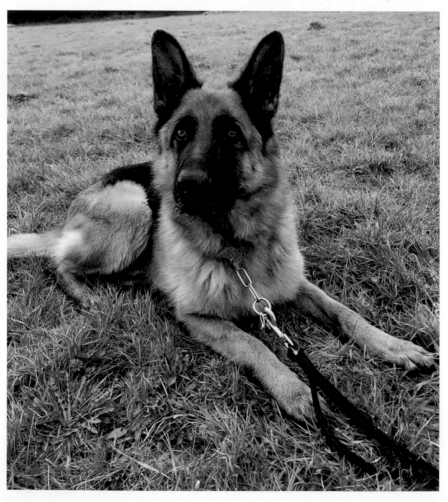

Reece Duffy January 2021.

Postscript

In this volume that has turned out rather larger than I had at first anticipated, I hope that within it I have given the reader something of interest and use, however small. Whether a new way of explaining an old truth, an old way of looking at something new or a new snippet of information altogether, its aim throughout has been to further the understanding and welfare of dogs. In turn, caring for their mental state and behaviour must be beneficial all round – to their families, friends and society at large. Dogs are so much part of our everyday lives that they have run the risk of becoming mundane. But we must not take them for granted. They deserve far better.

Setting aside the health and welfare implications for them, it is an insult to dogs either to be treated as fashion accessories or acquired purely for human social comfort (as during the current Covid-19 pandemic), to be picked up and discarded at a whim. It is humbling to realise the extent of their social intelligence and that they understand us and our emotions far better than we understand them. If our attentions are rejected, we cannot assume that they are in some way defective and non-representative of their species. The words of Ian Dunbar are indelibly imprinted on my memory: *'Touching a dog is a privilege to be earned'*. Everything is there in that one short phrase.

My first word was 'd-d-doggun!' much to my mother's amusement and my father's disappointment. In retrospect, it now seems that what began as a baby's eagerly awaited first word became a self-fulfilling prophecy.

A final anecdote:

A nurse was discharging a bitch spay of mine, which happened to be pure white. While she was explaining the necessary post-operative care, the owner noticed a red mark on top of the dog's head. Rather concerned and wondering if it was blood, she asked the nurse about it. The nurse replied, "Oh, it's nothing to worry about. That's where the vet kissed her!"

References

Baumgaertner, S., Mullan, D. C. J., and Main, H., 2016. Assessment of unnecessary suffering in animals by veterinary experts. *Veterinary Record*, 179, 307.

Bradshaw, J., 2010. Could empathy for animals have been an adaptation in the evolution of Homo?' *Animal Welfare*, 19.

Casey et al., 2014. Human directed aggression in domestic dogs – occurrence in difference contexts and risk factors. *Applied Animal Behaviour Science*, 152, 52–63.

Cooper, J., Cooper, M., 2018. What is veterinary forensic medicine and why is it important? *Veterinary Practice*. (https://veterinary-practice.com/article).

Csányi, V., 2006. *If Dogs Could Talk: Exploring of the Canine Mind*. North Point Press.

Drews, 1993. The concept and definition of dominance in animal behaviour. *Behaviour*, 125, 283–311.

Dugatkin, L. A., 2018. The silver fox domestication experiment. *Evolution: Education and Outreach*, 11, 16.

Evans, J. M. and White, K., 1997. *Doglopaedia: A Complete Guide to Dog Care*. Publisher Howell Book House.

Guo, K., Meints, K., Hall, C., Hall, S., and Mills, D., 2009. Left Gaze Bias in humans, Rhesus monkeys and domestic dogs. *Animal Cognition*, 12(3), 409–418.

Frederick, E. 2019. Humans have not just changed what dogs look like: we've altered the very structure of their brains, *Science*, September 2. www.sciencemag.org.

Hecht, E. E. et al., 2019. Significant neuroanatomical variation among domestic dog breeds. *Journal of Neuroscience*, 39, 7748–7758.

Horowitz, A., 2009. Disambiguating the "Guilty Look": Salient prompts to a familiar dog behaviour. *Behavioural Processes*, 81(3), 447–452.

House of Commons Environment, Food and Rural Affairs Committee, 2018. Controlling dangerous dogs Ninth Report of Session 2017–19, September 12.

Janssens et al., 2018. A new look at an old dog: Bonn-Oberkassel reconsidered. *Journal of Archaeological Science*, 92, 126–138.

Lord et al., 2020. The history of farm foxes undermines the animal domestication syndrome. *Trends in Ecology and Evolution*, 35(2), 125–136.

McGreevy, P., 2004, Correlation between retinal cell distribution and nose length, *Brain, Behaviour and Evolution*, 63, 13–22.

McGreevy, P. D., Wilson, B., Starling, M. J., and Serpell, J. A., 2018. Behavioural risks in male dogs with minimal lifetime exposure to gonadal hormones may complicate population-control benefits of desexing. *PLoS ONE*, 13(5), e0196284. https://doi.org/10.1371/journal.pone.0196284.

Mech, D., 1970. *The Wolf: Ecology and Behavior of an Endangered Species*. Publisher University of Minnisota.

Mech, D., 2008. Whatever happened to the term 'alpha wolf'? *International Wolf*, 18, 4.

Notari, L. and Mills, D., 2016. Is there a link between treatments with exogenous corti-costeroids and dog behaviour problems? *Veterinary Record*, 5, 179(18), 462.

O'Neill, D. et al., 2017. Demography and disorders of German Shepherd Dogs under primary veterinary care in the UK. *Canine Genetics and Epidemiology*, 4, 7.

Ostojic et al., 2015. Are owners' reports of their dogs' 'guilty look' influenced by the dogs' action and evidence of the misdeed? *Behavioural Processes*, 111, 97–100.

Overall, K., 2007. Working bitches and the neutering myth: Sticking to the science. *The Veterinary Journal*, 173, 9–11.

Pangal, S., 2019. Study on the activity budget of free-ranging dogs *BHARCS,* June 26. www. livesofstreeties.org.

Parsons, K. J. et al., 2020. Skull morphology diverges between urban and rural populations of red foxes mirroring patterns of domestication and macroevolution. *Proceedings of the Royal Society B: Biological Sciences*, 287, 20200763.

Positive Police Dogs. Available at: www.positivepolicedogs.wordpress.com.

Riggio, G. and Nonni, V., 2020. Pain or anxiety: The case of a 12-year-old German Shepherd. *Dog Behavior*, 1, 31–37.

Rowell, T. E., 1974. The concept of social dominance. *Behavioural Biology*, 11, 2.

Rugaas, T. E., 1997. On Talking Terms with Dogs: Calming Signals, *Legacy By Mail*, Carlsborg, WA.

Serpell, J., 2002. Anthropomorphism and anthropomorphic selection: Beyond the cute response. *Society and Animals*, 10(4), 437–454.

Shepherd, K., 2002. Development of Behaviour, social behaviour and communication in dogs in *BSAVA Manual of Canine and Feline Behavioural Medicine*, BSAVA.

Shepherd, K., 2007. Behavioural husbandry: The way to a client's heart. *Practice*, 29, 540–544.

Shepherd, K. and Mills, D., 2007. Animal training and behaviour in *BSAVA Textbook of Veterinary Nursing 4th edition*, BSAVA.

Shepherd, K., 2009. Behavioural medicine as an integral part of veterinary practice, in Debra F. Horwitz and Daniel S. Mills (Eds.) *BSAVA Manual of Canine and Feline Behavioural Medicine 2nd edition*, BSAVA, 3–6.

Shepherd, K., 2011. Animal training and behaviour in *BSAVA Textbook of Veterinary Nursing 5th edition*, BSAVA.

Shepherd, K., 2013. Teaching dog owners new tricks. *Veterinary Record*, 583–584.

Shepherd, K., 2017. The assessment of dogs for legal cases: A UK perspective, in Daniel Mills and Carri Westgarth (Eds.) *Dog Bites: A Multidisciplinary Perspective*. 5m Publishing.

Waller, B. et al., 2013. Paedomorphic expressions give dogs a selective advantage. *PLOS One*, 8, 12.

Zaczek, I., 2000. *Dogs – A Dog's Life in Art and Literature*. Cologne Germany: Taschen.

Index